DATE DUE

BORN TO DIE?

BORN TO DIE?
Deciding the Fate
of Critically Ill Newborns

EARL E. SHELP

THE FREE PRESS
A Division of Macmillan, Inc.
NEW YORK

Collier Macmillan Publishers
LONDON

Copyright © 1986 by The Free Press
          A Division of Macmillan, Inc.

All rights reserved. No part of this book may be reproduced
or transmitted in any form or by any means, electronic or
mechanical, including photocopying, recording, or by any
information storage and retrieval system, without permission
in writing from the Publisher.

The Free Press
A Division of Macmillan, Inc.
866 Third Avenue, New York, N.Y. 10022

Collier Macmillan Canada, Inc.

Printed in the United States of America

printing number
1 2 3 4 5 6 7 8 9 10

Library of Congress Cataloging-in-Publication Data

Shelp, Earl E.
  Born to die?

  Includes bibliographies and index.
    1. Infants (Newborn)—Diseases—Treatment—Moral and
ethical aspects.   2. Parent and child.   3. Euthanasia—
Moral and ethical aspects.   4. Infanticide—History.
I. Title.   [DNLM: 1. Abnormalities—therapy.
2. Decision Making.   3. Ethics, Medical.   4. Infant,
Newborn, Diseases—therapy.   5. Life Support Care.
6. Morals.   7. Parents.   WS 420 S544b]
RJ255.S37   1986   174'.24   85-20546
ISBN 0-02-929110-0

Contents

Preface

M<small>Y INTEREST</small> in the medical care of newborn infants began in 1979. What began as occasional conferences with the neonatologists, nurses, and social workers in a neonatal intensive care nursery has evolved gradually to become a regularly scheduled weekly activity in intermediate and intensive care units. During these meetings cases are presented. These are not meetings that directly result in treatment decisions. Rather, these are teaching conferences in which moral, medical, legal, and psychosocial features of particular patients are analyzed and discussed. This participation in the world of newborn medicine has enabled me to observe first-hand the drama that often attends the care of an infant born with severe congenital diseases or defects. I have come to conclude as a result of my observations and understandings of the moral dimensions of these cases that some are complex and perplexing to everyone intimately involved.

Simplistic answers and uniform responses to these instances of reproductive tragedy, I am convinced, simply are not morally justifiable or practical. What one may perceive from a distance to be morally required may be viewed differently from the midst of the dilemma itself. Thus, in this volume, which examines the ethics of neonatology, I unapologetically have tried to express representative intellectual and emotional components of the medical-moral decision-making process. In an effort to illustrate how these components can interact and their respective influence on decisions, I have included case studies at several points in the text. These reports have been altered to protect the identities of actual participants. Some cases are abbreviated, others are more comprehensively presented. The intentions for these cases are: (1) to highlight the relevance of the topic being discussed, (2) to representatively illustrate how the task of making medical-moral decisions for severely impaired or diseased newborns proceeds, and (3) to demonstrate that the perceived interest of the newborn is only one of several morally licit considerations in these situations.

The professional personnel with whom I work in several settings have welcomed me into their world. Nothing in this volume is intended to betray their confidence or to cast a shadow on men and women for whom I have profound respect. Similarly, I have come to admire the courage, patience, wisdom, and compassion that most parents exhibit as they cope with the birth of an impaired baby. It continues to be a privilege to struggle with parents and professionals to understand the moral choices that are open to them. I have learned from them all. These numerous experiences have helped to shape the views that are presented here.

This book is written for people concerned about moral dilemmas in the care of severely diseased or defective newborn infants. It is addressed to neonatologists, pediatricians, obstetricians, parents, social workers, nurses, clergy, and ethicists. Parts of the volume speak more directly to one audience than to others. It is hoped, however, that the analyses, expositions, and perspectives, as a whole, will enrich the understanding of all about the emotionally charged controversies that often attend treatment decisions for imperiled newborn infants. My focus is on the nursery and the decisions for or against treatment in that context. Questions regarding the allocation of national resources to the medical care and subsequent support of impaired newborns have been set aside. By setting these matters aside I do not mean to dismiss their relevance to clinical decisions. Surely the type and availability of supportive services from public and private agencies affect the range of options for any particular case. These factors are givens. They are not subject to change by the individuals responsible for making decisions regarding a particular infant's care. Decisions are made with a view toward these opportunities or constraints. The allocation of national resources to the treatment of newborns and to survivors with care needs stemming from neonatal diseases or defects merits a sustained moral and policy analysis. Changes may occur as a result of these analyses or in response to political pressures. It is not likely, however, that changes will take place quickly enough to significantly alter the options that may be chosen among in a particular case. It is for this reason, not because issues of macroallocation are not relevant or important, that these matters are bracketed in this volume. The interest here is on the immediate decisions and circumstances that frequently determine whether an infant lives or dies. I have intentionally avoided making judgments about the moral probity of any particular treatment decision. The reasons for this will become apparent as the reader progresses through the volume. The guidance provided here is procedural and substantive, but not specific for particular diagnoses. This is an empathic introduction to and reasoned analysis of moral questions related to the medical care of severely diseased or defective newborns. As such, I hope that it will be of service to everyone concerned about these matters.

A Preview

This moral exploration in neonatology is addressed to a general audience. It is especially directed to those key actors in the dramas that occur in newborn nurseries who actually evaluate options and make decisions that portend a life with handicap or an early death for a severely diseased or defective baby.

Readers hoping to find a manual that specifies what ought to be decided for newborn infants with particular diagnoses will be disappointed by this book. Such a volume conceivably could be written. It could provide general guidance but it could not, in my opinion, anticipate the exigencies of all actual or prospective cases.[1] Conceptual ethical, general clinical, and operational criteria, like those proposed by ethicist Robert Weir,[2] can be forwarded, but dilemmas persist. The problems of providing substance to the criteria and of rightly discerning, to the satisfaction of all concerned, how they should apply to specific cases would remain. Accordingly, the approach offered and defended here focuses first on who properly bears the burden and responsibility of making these ominous decisions, and second, on the discretion that these agents may properly exercise in discerning a morally good and right course. A form of guidance will be extended to parents, medical personnel, and policymakers in the process. However, the

guidance is more procedural than substantive. Substantive recommendations for specific categories of neonates would tend to be
mainly expressions of an author's biases, which may be only one of
several morally defensible options. This more limited agenda
seems required if one accepts the validity of a moral pluralism and
respects the autonomy of moral agents and moral communities
that constitute the fabric of the moral order.

The argument is based on three assumptions: first, that value is
attached to all human life but what specific moral duties persons
have toward every instance of human life is an unsettled issue; second, that decisions in the medical context are guided by the same
moral principles and rules utilized in other areas of human activity;
and third, that the moral order is pluralistic and that public policy
ought to be secular in nature. This methodological approach
honors the priority of principles and rules over utilitarian justifications for conduct, though consequences of decisions and actions
are considered relevant. The moral principles of autonomy, beneficence, and justice are pivotal to the positions advocated here and to
their justification. Thus, this study provides a conceptual and normative inquiry and perspective on a controversial zone of moral
choice. It articulates a view that maximizes morally acceptable
alternatives for families, health care personnel, and society in coping with newborn misfortune and tragedy.

A central concern of this study is the nature and limit of parental
authority with regard to the medical care of a child. The claim will
be advanced in Chapter 1 that parents normally are morally responsible to direct the care of their imperiled newborn infant. Insofar as their decisions are reasonable, they warrant respect by
care-providers. This proposition will be supported by interpretations of three moral principles seen to be relevant to the questions
of who decides and the range of concerns morally relevant to treatment decisions. This claim and its defense grows out of an understanding of the moral order as pluralistic, composed of numerous
individual moral communities which co-exist but, nevertheless,
embrace particular visions of the good, right, and wrong.

In order to place the contemporary discussion about the care of
defective newborns in perspective, Chapter 2 reviews the relation
of parent and child in custom, philosophy, religion, and law. It will
be shown that children basically have been valued in relation to
parents who have been primarily responsible and authorized to
prepare a child for independent existence within a particular social

order. Intrusions into the family unit or usurpations of parental authority by the state or other parties have been uncommon and of dubious justification, given the operative cultural and intellectual presuppositions regarding, and expectations for, the tasks of parenting.

The examination of parental responsibility and authority is extended in Chapter 3 with a perspective on the risks and responsibilities of parenting today. Among the risks is the chance that a pregnancy will end with the birth of a defective or impaired infant. Parental responses to this untoward event are varied. A trusteelike or quasi-trustee model of parental obligations and authority regarding child care will be proposed. It will be argued that this approach is consistent with historical precedents and can accommodate diverse particular moral judgments.

Parents are increasingly able to exercise responsibility for the medical care of severely ill or defective newborns because of the enhanced powers of medicine to intervene effectively to prolong life and lessen or correct limitations caused by diseases or defects. In Chapter 4, the rise of neonatology as a subspecialty within pediatric medicine will be traced and its performance will be evaluated. Neonatology will be described as a context in which competing interests may be expressed and negotiated. The necessity to make choices, in these situations of conflict, regarding whether and to what extent to intervene medically, may occasion a moral quandary in the decision to attempt rescue, let die, or terminate newborn life. The role of the neonatologist in situations where "hard choices" are required will be described as a "sustaining presence," cooperating with parents who express varying moral visions. Finally, arguments favoring physicians, hospital-based committees, or judges to make treatment decisions for imperiled newborns will be analyzed and found insufficient to unseat the strong presumption that parents properly bear this responsibility.

The process of making treatment decisions is analyzed in Chapter 5. Two approaches to determining what is morally required or allowed in these adverse circumstances will be evaluated. One approach decides moral duty on the basis of the status of newborn humans as persons and/or the likelihood that they will become persons in the moral sense of the word. The second approach bases moral duty on the value that life does and will have for the newborn and others, given the infant's condition and a belief that survival is possible. It will be argued that both methods of making treatment decisions express valid moral concerns. Further, it will be shown that there is potential for agreement and disagreement within and between both approaches. Finally, several proposals are made regarding how the task of making valid decisions might proceed.

Chapter 6 focuses on the forms that a morally acceptable response to neonatal misfortune may take. It will have been argued previously that defective infants, particularly those reasonably believed never able to become persons or attain a minimal level of independence, are subject to the almost exclusive authority of their parents to determine their medical care or lack of it. Destined by their diseases or defects to a severely impaired existence or a prolonged death, if life-supporting procedures are initiated and continued, these infants present a profound dilemma to care providers and the moral community: Should they be allowed to die, or should death be effected in a merciful manner? An answer to this question will be advanced through a survey of historical practices of infanticide and an analysis of the alleged moral distinction between killing and letting die. In addition, present practices with respect to those infants for whom death is judged an acceptable alternative to prolonged life will be described and compared to an alternative of mercifully assisting the death of newborn life.

The legal and policy implications of the proposals in this text are substantial. Chapter 7 reviews governmental efforts to intercede in a zone of decision making that heretofore has tended to be the nearly exclusive province of parents and physicians. Federal regulations and legislative proposals regarding medical treatment for anomalous newborns will be summarized, evaluated, and found to be ill-advised. The chapter concludes with an argument that the law can and should accept the proposition, which is also the thesis of this volume, that parents bear the burden and authority, except in rare instances, to decide the medical care of severely defective newborns in the light of their moral values, commitments, principles, and norms. In these specific instances, the interests of the state in infant life that would warrant intercession are held to be negligible.

The arguments and conclusions in this volume will be seen by some as outrageous, by others as controversial. My hope, however, is that they will be received by a larger readership as a reasonable and sensitive examination of a complex and perplexing realm of moral and medical decision making. After six years of experiencing the day-to-day tragedies of reproductive mishap as they unfolded in intermediate and intensive care neonatal nurseries, my aim in preparing this volume is not to compound the pain, suffering, and strife that can follow the birth of a severely impaired baby. Rather, my aim is to generate a greater empathy for the parents, physicians, nurses, social workers, and families who must face the brutal facts of reproductive mishaps and attempt to respond to them in a redemptive manner. Finally, and more importantly, my aim is to illuminate relevant issues, concepts, and concerns in a humane and intellectual light. Even if the arguments and conclusions are not universally accepted, which surely they will not be, perhaps the inquiry that they may engender will contribute to a more reasoned and complete airing of views and differences, which will lead to a greater mutual respect for our considered, and perhaps considerable, disagreements.

Many people have been of help to me in the preparation of this volume. Only a few can be specifically mentioned. My colleagues in neonatology, especially James Adams and Mike Speer, exercised much patience in helping me to understand the meaning and implications of relevant medical diagnoses. Baruch Brody, director of the Center for Ethics, where I work, encouraged me to address these issues in book form. Delores Smith labored many hours trying to read my writing in order to put the text on a word processor. Audrey Laymance assisted with the typing of rough drafts. Jay Jones, my research assistant, was of help from start to finish. Warren Reich introduced me to The Free Press. Laura Wolff, at The Free Press, provided editorial counsel. H. Tristram Engelhardt, Jr., Ronald H. Sunderland, Raymond S. Duff, Albert R. Jonsen, and J. Robert Nelson read the full manuscript, providing helpful criticisms and comments. David Hannah, Bill Smith, and Julian Byrd at Hermann Hospital; Harvey Richardson and the congregation of Kenwood Baptist Church; International Studies in Philosophy and Medicine, Inc., Al Parker, and Mrs. D. K. Poole in varying ways helped to underwrite the expenses associated with the research and preparation of the manuscript. Each of these people, and many others whose specific contribution has not been identified, should know of my gratitude. Without the generous assistance of each one this project would have been impossible to complete.

BORN TO DIE?

1

Introduction

MARY AND JOHN ARE in their sixth year of marriage. John is a salesman who travels around the state, often being away from home for weeks at a time. Mary is a waitress. They have a four-and–a-half-year-old son who is cared for by John's mother while Mary is at work. Despite the time that Mary and John are apart, they are devoted to each other and to their son. Their combined incomes allow them to live modestly.

During the thirty-first week of Mary's second pregnancy she gave birth to twin sons weighing 49 ounces (1,400 grams) and 50.4 ounces (1,440 grams) respectively. Both premature babies were diagnosed with Down syndrome, a condition characterized by distorted features and varying levels of mental retardation. Twin A, in addition to Down syndrome, was found to have other problems associated with prematurity, which were successfully treated. Twin A went home from the hospital within three weeks of birth. Twin B was not so fortunate. During the course of his hospitalization he developed multiple organ failure. He required surgery to remove part of the bowel, which did not function, and to repair a perforation of the colon. A tube had to be inserted into the heart to administer nutrients. He became ventilator dependent, required 100 percent oxygen, developed fluid in the lungs, and pneumonia. His blood pressure was supported by drugs. His kidneys failed. His liver did not function properly. Thus, over the course of two and a half months, this baby developed severe, life-

threatening disorders of the bowel, lungs, liver, heart, and kidneys. All of these events occurred independently of and in addition to having Down syndrome, which affected to an unknown
extent his future mental development. To maintain Twin B's life,
numerous medical interventions were required. Whether these
multiple interventions would save the baby's life was uncertain
to the neonatologists and other pediatric consultants. It appeared
to the neonatal team that death was imminent on three occasions,
but with intensive care the baby's condition was stabilized. However, even if Twin B survived, they could not predict with any
reasonable degree of certainty what level of special care, beyond
that usually required for Down syndrome patients, would be necessary because of the long-term consequences of his multiple
medical problems following birth.

Mary, and John from a distance, were very interested in the
condition and progress of this baby. Mary visited daily, John on
weekends when he was home. The hospital and medical bills
were being paid by insurance coverage from Mary's employment.
They wanted this baby to live but worried about the effect the
twins would have on their marriage and the future of their first
child. The parents felt that one baby with Down syndrome would
be a heavy burden, but two, and one with at least one disease of
every organ system, was feared to be more than they could bear.
After ten weeks of watching Twin B deteriorate while the intensity of care was steadily increasing, they began to wonder if their
insistence that "everything be done" was justified. Would it be
better for Twin B if they withdrew, or at least not start additional,
"heroic" measures and allowed "nature to take its course"?
Would it be better for them as marital partners, for Twin A, and
their healthy son, if Twin B were allowed to die now without
further invasive efforts to defeat what appeared to be an inevitable death? Would it be morally permissible to intend the death
of Twin B by withdrawing one or more of the medical interventions that sustained his fragile existence? Could they and the physicians do so legally?

The sort of moral, legal, and medical dilemmas that Mary and
John faced are shared by many parents of severely defective or
diseased newborns and pediatricians specializing in their care
(neonatologists). Consider one more case. Terri was born to a
twenty-three–year–old woman. This was her fourth pregnancy—
the first pregnancy ended in miscarriage, the second resulted in

a stillbirth, and the infant born from the third died within six hours of delivery. The current pregnancy ended with the premature delivery (twenty-seven weeks) of a very low birth weight (21.9 ounces—625 grams) female infant. Soon after admission to intensive care, Terri was found to have severe bleeding in the brain (Grade 4 bilateral intraventricular hemorrhage) complicated by a buildup of fluids in the head (posthemorrhagic hydrocephalus). A computerized picture of the skull (CT scan) revealed a "bizarre brain anatomy," a picture that was "mostly hole," indicating that very little brain tissue remained undamaged. The baby's neurological problems were such that it was believed that neither spinal taps nor the surgical placement of a shunt to drain excess fluid from the head would represent a net benefit because of the probable complications of either procedure. This meant that needles had to be inserted through the baby's skull every two days to decrease fluid pressure in the head.

Terri also had chronic lung disease. She could not breathe on her own, so for five months she had a tube down her throat. Her trachea had become so scarred and narrow that if the tube were removed she would be unable to breathe. Her airway was too small for sufficient air to pass. A tracheostomy could bypass this problem, but it would necessitate her remaining in the hospital for probably another seven months while she grew to a size where she could be managed at home. Her general prognosis would be unaffected by this procedure—her chronic lung disease would not be cured and her brain damage would not be lessened. The extent of her brain damage suggested that she would have cerebral palsy and/or significant intellectual or mental impairments; she was reasonably expected to be profoundly neurologically impaired if she survived.

Both of Terri's parents worked. They were young and desperately wanted to start a family. Terri's mother would visit regularly but say very little to the doctors and nurses. Her father also visited, took Terri's picture, and read passages from the New Testament to her. The parents were sensitive to the serious nature of Terri's medical problems, but they were careful never to ask the neonatologists a question that could bring a pessimistic answer. They maintained a steady optimism regarding Terri's future. No frustration was ever expressed to the neonatal team. Her father consulted with the physicians regarding Terri's care and progress. He was told of each change in her condition and treat-

ment as it occurred. He often spoke of his desire for Terri to survive because "she lets me feel like a father."

The neonatal team questioned the wisdom of performing the
tracheostomy in light of Terri's neurological and pulmonary prognoses. Her care had become what they described as "therapeutically ridiculous," meaning that the intensity of care required to
maintain her life was "grossly disproportionate to the expected
outcomes." Further, the neonatal team was not certain that the
parents ever understood the full meaning of what had been told
to them in bits and pieces regarding the level of care Terri would
require outside of the hospital and the severity of her neurological
deficits. The team's sense of futility was heightened by the work
load in the intensive care unit: The ICU was filled to capacity
(twenty-three beds). In fact, it was frequently over capacity, with
care being given to twenty-six newborns. Other newborns who
could be expected to benefit more than Terri from intensive care
had to be referred elsewhere for treatment because there was no
space, personnel, or equipment available. The neonatologists
were in a quandary. They decided to speak frankly with Terri's
parents about her prognosis. They hoped that the parents would
decide to ask for a decreased level of care, which would probably
result in Terri's death, an end, in their judgment, that was in the
baby's best interest. For five months, the neonatologists had done
all they could to reverse or stabilize Terri's condition but to no
avail. They simply could not see the point of continuing, either
for Terri, her parents, themselves, or the newborns who were denied care because no resources were available.

Terri's parents listened carefully to all they were told. They
were torn in two directions. Terri was not the baby they expected
but she was their baby now, though her survival was uncertain
even with continued intensive care. They had tried to have a baby
three times before and Terri represented the most success yet.
They were not inclined to let her go unless they were convinced
beyond any doubt that it was in her interest. On the other hand,
they recognized the burden of care Terri would present if she survived. Further, and more importantly, they were not certain that
life would be of any value to Terri if the medical prognosis proved
accurate. They were concerned about her pain and suffering. They
did not want to force her to live if life would be meaningless to
her. The right decision was not immediately clear to them. Should

they ask that Terri's care be maintained in order to maximize her chance to survive regardless of the quality of life she would have? Should they ask that Terri be allowed to die because continued life was not in her interests and/or theirs? Should the neonatologists effectively make the decision by altering Terri's care on the basis of their estimate of the net value of their interventions for Terri and in light of their desire to allocate scarce resources to produce the greatest net benefits?

In the past, parents and physicians, indeed nearly everyone, undertood these unfortunate situations as private tragedies. Parents and physicians were trusted to do what was "best." Today, however, cases like these and the medical decisions they generate are matters of public inquiry and debate. When forced to make difficult decisions that mean life or death for a newborn, parents and physicians tend to be troubled by the awesomeness of the decision. Their anxiety does not stem solely from a desire to make a "right" decision. It is generated as well by an awareness, particularly among physicians, that a third party or governmental agent may not only seek to override their decision, but may also bring civil or criminal charges against them. Personal misfortune has been transformed into an arena of public oversight. The benevolent commitments of parents and physicians to newborn infants are no longer regarded in some quarters as dependable safeguards of the welfare and best interests of newborns with severe defects, or debilitating or life-threatening diseases. Accordingly, efforts have been made to limit or deny parents in concert with physicians the freedom to decide what is morally and medically proper.

The widely publicized case that precipitated a vigorous federal effort to invade the precincts of medical decision making for defective newborns involved a male infant born April 15, 1982, in Bloomington, Indiana. Like the twins discussed above, "Baby Doe" had Down syndrome as well as a condition in which his esophagus was not connected to his stomach (tracheoesophageal fistula), which made oral feeding impossible. There were also indications of a heart defect (possible aortic coarctation). The first condition could have been surgically repaired immediately. The second condition could have been surgically repaired later. The parents, with court approval, refused surgical treatment, food, and water. The baby was given medicine as needed for pain and restlessness. His parents visited and held him frequently until he died on his sixth day of life.[1]

Less than a month following this case, the Department of Health and Human Services sent a "Notice to Health Care Providers" threatening hospitals with a loss of federal funding if newborns were allowed to die without medical treatment or nutrition "because of the existence of a concurrent handicap, such as Down syndrome."[2] This notice was the first of several regulatory and legislative efforts, to mandate life-saving interventions for all newborns regardless of handicap. Whereas before, parents and physicians were basically at liberty to make treatment decisions that were responsive to the facts of an infant's condition and the values and circumstances of its family, this pattern of individualized decision making was placed in jeopardy following Baby Doe.

It should be observed in passing, however, that the practice of allowing severely defective newborns to die neither began, nor was first announced, with "Baby Doe." For example, neonatologists Raymond S. Duff and A. G. M. Campbell wrote about their experiences in a special care nursery in 1973—nine years earlier. Their article, published in the New England Journal of Medicine, reported that 14 percent (43 out of 299) of the deaths or their timing in the special care nursery of the Yale–New Haven Hospital between January 1, 1970, through June 30, 1972, were "associated with discontinuance or withdrawal of treatment."[3] All of these babies had some form of severe impairment that, in the judgment of parents and physicians, made their prognosis for a meaningful life extremely poor or hopeless. On this basis, these newborns were allowed to die. Yet this controversial report did not provoke the sort of governmental action that followed the death of Baby Doe. One can only speculate why. It seems reasonable, however, to imagine that the increased influence of the so-called right-to-life movement and the presence of a sympathetic administration in Washington were important factors. The debate that has accompanied the legalization of abortion now promises to attend with similar intensity parental decisions against medical interventions that might prolong the lives of severely defective or diseased newborns. The moral pluralism that stands behind disagreements regarding abortion is similarly reflected in diverse viewpoints regarding decisions that foresee and/or intend the deaths of certain impaired neonates.

Moral Communities and Moral Principles

The diversity of the moral community is amply demonstrated by disagreement regarding the morality of abortion. This issue, perhaps more than any other, indicates that moral opinion in the United States is divided about certain issues. I do not mean to suggest that only now has American society become morally pluralistic, or that the issue of abortion is the first evidence of its moral diversity. Rather, the issue of abortion has displayed the social implications of a moral pluralism in ways that lead some to embrace the mutual respect it entails and others to resist the advent of a perceived "normlessness." The situation is one of multiple moral visions, existing side by side, offering varying perspectives, worldviews, and approaches to understandings of right and wrong.

Though there probably never has been a time in which moral differences among people did not coexist, the climate is such now that these differences are publicly sanctioned and protected. Individual judgments regarding abortion, artificial insemination, in vitro fertilization, contraception, sterilization, and homosexuality, to identify only a few disputed issues, tend to reflect the wisdom of the particular moral community with which one identifies, either religious or philosophical. Thus, the moral order is comprised of subcommunities of utilitarians, humanists, Jews, Protestants, Roman Catholics, Moslems, atheists, and professions, among others, all of whom often express distinct moral viewpoints. The differences that mark contemporary moral reflection, in the words of theologian Ted Peters, "cannot be washed away; they cannot be uprooted or overcome, absorbed or ignored, assimilated or dissipated. They are an indelible characteristic of modern life."[4]

Such an entrenchment of moral pluralism has led Alasdair MacIntyre, a philosopher, to observe that "There seems to be no rational way of securing moral agreement in our culture."[5] If the moral debate about abortion is an indication of the prospects for consensus regarding other disputable issues in medical practice, including the nontreatment of defective newborns, MacIntyre's observation may be correct, agreement may not be reached. However, a failure to establish a single morality, whether rooted in philosophy or religion, may not be a cause for despair. In a society founded on the premise that mature persons have a right to ar-

ticulate and choose among competing philosophies, religions, and
moralities, a diversity of life-styles, beliefs, and moral sentiments
should come as no surprise. Rather than viewing a flourishing of
defensible moralities as an indication that somehow moral agents
and society have lost their way, perhaps we should celebrate the
variety of moral visions as a safeguard against self-righteousness
and unjust intolerance. In addition, discontent with our differences may occasion a dialogue that leads to greater mutual understanding, and possibly consensus. Critical inquiry and
reflection about the nature of morality, and its multiple expressions, may lead to a clearer comprehension of the concepts, principles, and values that constitute its core substance. Such a
clarification would have merit, even if we fail to resolve the issues
that divide us. Perhaps the suspicion, distrust, and disrespect that
frequently stem from ignorance of another's rational, though different, opinion will subside and be replaced by a rising tolerance
and mutual respect based on a greater understanding of reasonable differences.

There seems to be a tendency in discussions about morality
to focus on those issues about which there is intense disagreement. Indeed, it is at these junctures that the pluralistic character
of the moral community is richly displayed. An observer of these
sometimes heated exchanges might conclude that agreement in
any area of life is beyond the reach of the disputants. This conclusion, however, would be mistaken. There are matters about
which people of diverse moral commitments agree. Indeed, there
must be certain agreements for human society, as it is now known,
to exist. These basic agreements constitute a minimum common
morality without which social organization and cooperation
would be either severely restricted or impossible. As importantly,
these agreements express certain moral values, ideals, goals, and
commitments that are widely shared despite particular differences. This common morality is the cement that holds the broad
moral community together. It specifies those behaviors that are
expected, those duties that should be performed, those obligations that should be acknowledged, and those rules that should
be observed.[6] The community defined by these basic agreements
and rules is referred to in this volume as the general or broad
moral community, the structure of which is found in its procedural agreements. Within these procedural agreements, persons
are free to fashion, discover, and pursue concrete and relative

views of the good life. They also are free to associate with others to constitute a subgroup or particular moral community within society to pursue some shared or mutually agreed upon values or ends. The basis of association, for example, may be certain religious beliefs (e.g., Mormonism and Catholicism) or certain professional commitments (e.g., medicine).

These particular moral communities in a pluralistic society are justified insofar as they do not violate the rules and agreements that give definition or identity to the social organization.[7] For example, there are rules prohibiting murder, assault, and theft. These rules reflect our collective sense about the inviolability of a person's body and property. The validity of these rules is not debated (in usual circumstances). People are expected to act in accord with them. An unjustified breach, whether by an individual or group, is not tolerated. If these basic rules are not enforced, it is believed that the security and moral integrity of the community and persons would be seriously jeopardized. Thus, rules to protect the physical being of persons and their property are endorsed by particular moral communities and the persons who constitute the general moral community. People may disagree with these basic rules, but they may not violate them with impunity.

There are other areas in life where rules governing individual or community choices are not warranted. These are areas where consensus is not necessary to social intercourse (e.g., style of dress) or where moral and other arguments are such that agreement may not be reached (e.g., homosexuality). In the first instance, the matter of one's attire is too trivial to warrant social control or require social agreement. In the second instance, homosexual relationships, in and of themselves, do not disrupt social peace. Judgments about them tend to reflect the moral sense of particular communities that may or may not be shared by other communities. In short, opinions of homosexuality tend to be matters of relative moral value and personal taste. Given the nature of these differences *and* the absence of a threat to social order, homosexual relations are not proper subjects for social control. Relative judgments about the morality of consensual homosexual, heterosexual, or bisexual relations will reflect the pluralism of the general moral community. Agreement and rules governing sexual relations are not necessary to protect the common values, ideals, goals, and commitments that transcend particular moral communities and identify us as a people. This is an area where personal freedom is primary and diversity should be respected. This is an area where our moral pluralism is manifested.

The care and treatment of newborn infants is also a context in which the moral pluralism of American society is brought into sharp focus. The birth of a baby that is premature, of low or very low birth weight, severely malformed, impaired, or diseased is an occasion for sorrow. It can turn expectation into disappointment, hope into despair, and joy into misery. Whereas in the past these infants were beyond the grasp of medicine to rescue, today the power of neonatal medicine to save has been enhanced to the point where serious questions are raised within professional and lay circles about the wisdom of doing so. The disparate judgments regarding this important and emotional issue, and the arguments offered to justify them, indicate that particular moral communities have loyalties and understandings of concepts and values that can lead "good" people to different choices. In an environment where definitive guidance is lacking about what is morally required in response to the birth of a defective newborn, decision makers should be free to express their reasonable moral convictions. Some may choose to prolong life, where this is possible; some may elect to allow the infant to die; and others may decide to directly end the newborn's life. Whichever choice is made, particular conceptual and value presuppositions are expressed.

The birth of a defective newborn is an event that may pose a moral dilemma to those individuals, especially parents and physicians, responsible for its care. For in these instances the presumptions that continued existence is an unqualified good and that actions intended to prolong life are morally required are sometimes cast into reasonable doubt. Guidance acceptable to every segment of the moral community simply is not available.

This volume examines some of the concepts, values, principles, and metaphors relevant to situations of reproductive tragedy. By so doing, the thesis that parents are the proper decision makers in these adverse situations and that their reasonable choices warrant respect will be articulated and defended. Two basic arguments will support this thesis: (1) that human neonates are not moral agents or persons in the same sense as normal older humans, and (2) that continued existence of a severely diseased or defective newborn may constitute a burden on it or on others sufficient to render life-extending interventions morally optional. These arguments are put forth with the assumption that the state should adopt a position of impartiality with respect to diverse but licit (reasonable) parental choices regarding the care of severely defective newborns. Within this sort of environment, particular moral traditions can be embraced and pursued in security. Parents, neonatologists, pediatric consultants, nurses, and social workers, who constitute the caring matrix of neonatal medicine, can hold diverse individual and professional judgments about what action is morally indicated. In this sense, neonatal medicine is a microcosm of the moral community in general. Deeply held convictions about one's moral duty in these instances may or may not be shared by those who attend these young lives, and the task of decision making may incite disagreement, even conflict. Nevertheless, in a society where pluralism is the reality, and where a diversity of moral views is commonplace, even celebrated, reasonable parental decisions regarding the destiny of a defective newborn merit the respect of others, even those who dissent and see the situation in a different moral light. This is not to say, however, that dissenters are obliged to cooperate or perform actions that are believed by them to be morally wrong.

Certainty, either of the moral or medical variety, is a scarce commodity in that segment of newborn medicine where ''hard cases'' require ''hard choices.'' Where the good and the right are not clear, humility and not arrogance seems appropriate. Where moral convictions that guide in other situations seem to collapse in the face of the challenge posed by a defective newborn, self-righteousness has no place. Where moral differences are common, persuasion and not intimidation is the proper means of change. Where valid moral sentiments are numerous, legislation or regulation to establish a single moral view constitutes an offense against free choice, which is valued in and protected by the moral community.

The case reports with which this chapter began illustrate how decisions of profound moral significance may be forced upon parents and medical personnel by the birth of a severely diseased or defective newborn. As the frontiers of neonatal medicine are pushed unremittingly toward the rescue of more infants who heretofore would have died, moral, medical, and policy dilemmas are generated that call for fresh interpretations and applications of the received traditions in order to find our way. Despite the

complex circumstances and the potentially awesome consequences (death or severely impaired life), decisions are required.
Moral and nonmoral (e.g., social services) resources are called
upon for guidance and information. Options are identified. Justifications are examined. Judgments are made. From a moral point
of view, three principles appear particularly relevant to so-called
life or death decisions in neonatology: self-determination or autonomy, beneficence, and justice. It is important for the reader to
understand the author's interpretation of these principles in order to appreciate how they inform the conclusions that are
reached. The approach offered here does not lead to a determination of what ought or ought not be done in any given case.
Rather, it seeks to protect the expression of diverse moral perspectives so as to enable moral agents to hold that a particular
judgment or action is wrong but nevertheless within the right of
the alleged erring party to decide or do.

Principle of Autonomy

The principle of self-determination or autonomy in the context of
neonatology cannot apply to a newborn infant, who is not self-
determining. Rather, it applies to parents or others designated to
make decisions in behalf of an imperiled infant. The principle of
self-determination, or respect for the autonomy of persons, provides prima facie protection of the choices and actions of autonomous agents. It promotes freedom as a value and functions to
constrain interference with the autonomous actions of moral
agents.[8] An autonomous decision or action is grounded in one's
own values and beliefs, based on adequate information that is
comprehended, and not determined by internal or external factors that compel the decision or action. In short, the principle of
self-determination enhances the freedom or liberty of present
moral agents. It promotes the ideas of self-governance, freedom
of choice, and personal responsibility for individual decisions and
behaviors. It protects privacy and the rights of a person to determine his or her own life or property without specifying what
choices or actions should be embraced.[9] This is not to say that a
freely chosen action is always morally acceptable or in accord with
other moral principles, e.g., murder. If one's actions, even though
freely chosen, harm another moral agent without that agent's

consent, then those actions do not warrant respect and may be controlled by force if necessary (e.g., self-defense against assault). In these sorts of situations the prima facie protection of the principle of self-determintion yields to or is overridden by the principle of nonmaleficence, which imposes a prima facie duty not to wrong or inflict an evil on a nonconsenting person.

Neonates are in no way autonomous. They are totally dependent on more mature humans for the necessities of life. They are incapable of internalizing values or beliefs. They lack the rational capacities to comprehend facts or make choices. Rather than being self-determining, they are totally determined by the choices and actions of others, principally their parents. Thus, if the principle of self-determination or autonomy is relevant to or provides moral guidance in situations of reproductive misfortune, it would seem to apply most properly to those individuals customarily responsible for an infant's care and nurture—the parents.

The argument for parents as the appropriate persons to determine the interests, medical and nonmedical, of a diseased or anomalous newborn will be developed fully in the chapters that follow. This initial affirmation of parental authority and responsibility rests on certain beliefs about the character of the parents' relationship with the newborn infant. My presumption is that parents establish a bond with the infant during pregnancy and at birth. This bond of love usually disposes parents to have an interest in the infant's welfare, which takes the typical form of doing everything possible to prolong the infant's life. This desire for the imperiled infant to survive tends to carry with it a willingness to provide the care and support that the infant will require. This desire—characterized as benevolent disposition, presumption for treatment, and readiness to live with the consequences—would seem to apply to parents more readily than to other decision makers who have no bond with the infant. This appears particularly true with regard to living with the final decision. It seems unlikely that nonbonded surrogates would be prepared to personally provide ongoing care for a sick or handicapped child. Thus, the relationship parents have with their infant is not the same as the one a stranger would be expected to have. This difference, in my opinion, is sufficient at this stage of our inquiry to support a strong presumption that parents have a greater authority and responsibility than others to make treatment decisions. Arguments related to the community of interests between parents and newborn, the personal commitment of parents to the newborn, and respect for the integrity of the family unit strengthen the presumption for parents and weaken the claim of others to fill this role, all things being equal. Respect for the autonomy of the family, therefore, ought to support a presumption in favor of parental authority and create a presumption in favor of the parents' decision.[10]

As stated earlier, there is a presumption at the birth of a defective newborn that life-sustaining interventions will be undertaken. This presumption reflects the value that is conferred on newborn human life. It also reflects a desire to prolong life for a sufficient length of time in order to gather the information relevant to making an informed decision about how to proceed. It is then the responsibility of the parents, once this information is understood, to make a reasonable decision regarding the treatment or nontreatment of their severely diseased or defective newborn. Parents ought not to be required to make the objectively most reasonable decision or the decision preferred by a majority of people.[11] Their decision in these situations must be one that is reasonable,[12] and it should warrant the respect of others. The parents' decision ought not to be overridden because it is disliked by neighbors, friends, or family or different from that which others would do in their place.

The standard of reasonableness establishes the limits of parental autonomy or discretion to determine an imperiled newborn's fate. It is a standard commonly used in medicine and law. It is a standard of conduct for areas of action that require some measure of discretion. Reasonable conduct is allowed where it is impossible to specify behavior for all conceivable situations. These are situations where clear and absolute guidance is not available, where "judgment calls" that balance interests are appropriate. The standard of reasonableness in this type of circumstance expresses some measure of confidence that the relevant persons will use their knowledge and skill to act in a proper manner to achieve ends that maximize benefits and minimize harms.

Discretion is clearly sanctioned by the standard of reasonableness. It should not be inferred, however, that the content of reasonable is purely subjective. Reasonableness is not synonymous with expediency or conduct based on whim, fancy, or caprice. Rather, reasonable conduct is that which nonideological observers could consider fit and fair *in light of the circumstances and not illegitimate in view of the end attained.* Thus, on the one hand, the standard is external; it expresses what society demands of a person. It is not reducible to a particular actor's idiosyncratic notion of what is proper. On the other hand, it allows for a balancing of the probability and gravity of risk or harm against the value or good the actor seeks to advance. Further, the standard takes into consideration the circumstances and the capacity of the agent to meet identified risks. As a standard of conduct, the "reasonable person" is an ideal figure who does what society would expect and allow in adverse or risky situations where clear and convincing prescriptions for conduct are not available. This ideal person, it should be noted, is permitted in law human shortcomings and weaknesses that his or her community will accept in light of the circumstances.[13]

Consider the legal standard of reasonableness with respect to negligence in medicine. Reasonable medical conduct is that which exhibits the skill and learning commonly possessed by members of the profession who are in good standing. If a physician fails to perform at this level of competence, he or she may be liable for the harm that results to a patient. The law acknowledges that in certain situations medical opinion is divided about what is the best or better course of treatment. In these circumstances, the physician is judged by the tenets of the school of medicine of which he or she is a member. "School" here is understood as a recognized body of knowledge, with definite principles of practice, and accepted by at least a respectable minority of the profession. For example, there is disagreement within the medical profession about the treatment of anginal pain. Some physicians prefer to treat these chest pains, which stem from constricted blood flow through the coronary arteries, with medication. Others favor coronary bypass surgery. In short, the current standard for reasonable medical practice seems to be what is customary and usual in the profession, while recognizing that the profession does not, in every instance, speak in a single voice. The law allows professionals, by relying on this test, to define its own standard of conduct. This allowance reflects the respect the law has for the profession of medicine. It also reflects a reluctance to overburden practitioners with liabilities based on uneducated judgments.[14]

It seems proper to utilize reasonableness as the standard of conduct for parents confronted by a severely diseased or defective newborn. The cases specifically referred to here are those where

scholars in ethics and medical authorities disagree among and between themselves about what is right in light of the condition of
the infant and the circumstances. And public opinion about these
cases is still divided. In short, there is no medical, moral, or social
consensus about what conduct is required. A decision to treat or
not to treat tends to be reflective of a recognized moral tradition
whose guidance is respected in other areas of life. A policy that
extends respect for particular moral traditions or moral communities to the context of neonatology seems warranted. First, it
would undergird the traditional authority and responsibility of
parents to decide the care of their children. Second, it would be
supportive of the value given to the integrity of the family unit.
And last, the standard would not overburden the principals with
intrusions into areas where clear and convincing guidance is lacking. Understood in this fashion, the reasonableness standard for
the parental role in these circumstances of reproductive tragedy
is similar to the standard of conduct applied to other roles where
discretion is a crucial element.

Reasonableness, as such, becomes a community standard that
establishes the boundaries of discretion for parents in these particular circumstances. It acknowledges that there are risks or evils
to be managed. But more important, it implies that it is impractical, or perhaps impossible, to specify how to do so without first
hand knowledge of the facts and the circumstances. The community to which the standard refers includes parents and relevant bystanders (physicians, nurses, hospital social workers) who
are positioned to attend to and make critical decisions for imperiled newborns. What is customarily expected of parents with regard to normal newborns may be *un*reasonable in situations where
the newborn is not and predictably never will be normal. The
facts of the latter cases are sufficiently different to alter expectations of proper parental conduct.[15]

Judgments of reasonableness will depend on the facts of each
case and the options or ends that are plausibly attainable. Procedures could be instituted to facilitate making reasonable judgments. But procedures designed to predetermine or prejudice the
decision would undermine the standard. Procedures that might
enhance the prospect that a reasonable decision will be made by
parents, and which would not necessarily prejudice their judgment, might include: (1) assurances that accurate information has
been provided and understood; (2) a brief period of delay after

which the initial decision is affirmed; (3) provision of consultants as requested by parents; and (4) making the infant available for adoption during the time between the initial decision against treatment and its affirmation. None of these procedures would appear to limit the discretion of the parents. Similarly, they do not imply a presumption of unreasonableness or irresponsibility. This sort of process of making and implementing decisions plausibly would enhance the prospect that a reasonable decision would be made without limiting in advance parental discretion or authority. In situations where the parents make one of several possible reasonable decisions, any effort to impose an alternative, according to the arguments that have been advanced, would bear the burden of justification.

It should be clear from the above that the reasonableness standard does, in fact, place limits upon parental discretion. Instances in which parental refusal of medical treatment for an imperiled newborn would be unreasonable include: (1) where there is a clear social consensus about the net benefit of the intervention, e.g., vaccinations;[16] (2) where medical experts agree that intervention is nonexperimental and appropriate, e.g., antibiotics for acute bacterial infection[17] (not only would antibiotics be simple and effective, it is difficult to imagine what values and beliefs, except those held by certain religious groups, would argue against their use);[18] (3) where nonintervention would result in an otherwise avoidable death, e.g., blood transfusion; (4) where the expected result is a strong chance for a normal and a healthy life,[19] e.g., surgical repair of a minor heart defect; and (5) where failure to treat would materially increase the risk of serious bodily harm,[20] e.g., prolonged disregard of signs of oxygen insufficiency (blue color). Newborns with conditions and in circumstances like these should be treated despite the parental refusal.

Instances in which parental refusal of treatment would be reasonable include: (1) where there is no proven procedure or where there is conflicting medical advice,[21] e.g., Trisomy 13 and bleeding in the brain (Grade 4 bilateral intraventricular hemorrhage), respectively; (2) where there is less than a high probability that the result of treatment will be a normal or near normal life,[22] e.g., any condition in addition to neurological damage that has a high probability of profound impairment with no chance of cure; (3) where intervention would be futile,[23] e.g., birth weight below viability; and (4) where treatment would impose a grave burden on

the infant or others,[24] e.g., multiple surgeries to prolong a vegetative existence and where treatment would prolong life for only
days or weeks but would incur a financial debt that would severely restrict the family's opportunities. Newborns with conditions and in circumstances relevantly like these should not be
treated against the parents' wishes.

If parents request treatment in cases where medical intervention is futile or would impose a grave burden on the infant, as
defined above, it can justifiably be refused. If the treatment would
impose a grave burden only on the family, it could be given. Parents should be free to bear these burdens but it is not clear that
they have a responsibility to do so. (More will be said about this
in the discussions of the principles of beneficence and justice.) In
situations other than those listed here, the presumption could be
that parental decisions to treat a diseased or defective newborn
are reasonable.

These examples indicate some limits of parental discretion in
terms of the standard of reasonableness. There may be circumstances where it is not appropriate or feasible to defer to parental
judgments during the medical care of an imperiled newborn. For
example, parents are absent, parents are incompetent to make an
informed decision (e.g., unable to understand the facts or options), parental decision is unreasonable as defined above, when
there are events that were not foreseen which require an immediate response and for which there has been no advance parental
instruction, when there is an irresolvable disagreement between
the parents, and when a parental decision would require a care
provider to violate standards of professional practice, law, or conscience.

Clearly the focus here has been on the role of the parents in
these unfortunate circumstances, and more will be said in Chapter 4 about the role of the neonatologists and other professionals
in these settings. But it should be mentioned now that physicians
and nurses have a duty, according to my argument, to review
parental decisions to treat or not to treat a diseased or defective
newborn. As representatives of the patient's and society's interests in these matters, they should request a further review by the
appropriate authority (courts) when a parental decision seems
foolish, malicious, or unreasonable.

Parents, according to this expanded interpretation of the principle of autonomy, are presumed to have the authority and re-

sponsibility of making treatment decisions regarding their critically ill newborn. Their decision needs only to be reasonable in order to warrant respect by others. The standard of reasonableness limits the discretion of parents without stipulating what the decision should be. A more exact delineation of reasonable and unreasonable decisions than that provided above would subvert the discretion that wisdom dictates for complex circumstances in which the good and right are not readily and compellingly apparent. Similarly, the gravity to the infant of the burden of treatment, or to others as a result of treatment, sufficient to defeat a presumption for treatment, is properly subject to the same standard of reasonableness. This position acknowledges the traditional responsibility and authority of parents to determine the best interests of their children, giving family values and beliefs precedence over societal or other individually held values, which have no sustainable claim to moral superiority. And the burden on others that treatment portends can be taken into account. This initial defense of the authority of parents to refuse medical care for severely impaired infants will be buttressed by arguments throughout the remainder of this volume. It will be extended in Chapter 6 to propose that parents may reasonably and rightfully decide that the infant's life may be terminated by direct means.

Principle of Beneficence

The second principle relevant to these tragic circumstances is the principle of beneficence.[25] Whereas the principle of self-determination guards a moral agent's freedom to choose among and act within competing moral visions, the principle of beneficence provides substance to the moral life. It sets a general policy without specifying its exact content. In general, the principle articulates a "duty to help others further their important and legitimate interests."[26] In short, it summons moral agents to "do to others their good."[27] As intuitively appealing as these formulations sound, it is by no means settled within a moral pluralism what another's "interest" is, or what is his or her "good."[28] Any specific determination of "best interest" or "good" will be expressed in terms of the vision of a particular moral community. Thus, only within particular moral communities where commitments, major values, and visions are shared is one likely to find agreement with regard to the substance of interest or good intended by the principle of beneficence. Similarly, only within particular moral communities will the limits of one's moral obligation to benefit another likely be agreed upon.[29]

The notion that the general moral community has a unified concrete vision of the good, the good life, or the life worth living is no longer held in modern Western societies.[30] It is increasingly futile to appeal to such a notion as a shared basis for moral reasoning, as justification for a given act, or as justification for establishing one view of the good life over another competing view. Accompanying the decline of a unifying, concrete conception of the good, there has been an increased emphasis on the importance and adequacy of individual or personal conceptions of the good as a starting point of moral dialogue. These more individualistic notions are generally viewed as more limited in scope and authority, but important nonetheless to the moral life and a necessary consideration in moral judgment. Western democratic societies have deemphasized the preservation and promotion of the corporate good as an overriding value. Instead, the preservation and promotion of individual concrete views of the good life, which may benefit corporate life, enjoys superior status.[31]

This inverted order of priorities can rest on any number of premises. For example, one could argue that the good of and for an individual is more concrete, less abstract, than the good of and for society. Further, it could be held that the good of and for an individual is more subject to being known and less subject to diverse renderings than the good of and for society.[32] One could also argue, along the lines of John Stuart Mill, that a preference for plural individual goods results in a greater gain for all than an establishment of a single concrete view of the good. For Mill, ''mankind are greater gainers by suffering each other to live as seems good to themselves than by compelling each to live as seems good to the rest.''[33] His appreciation for individual freedom did not rest only on his estimate of a beneficial result to all. More accurately, his was an appreciation of liberty itself and a qualified affirmation of the individual. He wrote, ''If a person possesses any tolerable amount of common sense and experience, his own mode of laying out his existence is the best, not because it is the best in itself, but because it is his own mode.''[34]

An environment where many perceptions of the good or of the life worth living are respected can be quite dynamic. There is potential for agreement and conflict between moral agents and communities. The situation can become even more diverse when it is recognized that individual perceptions tend to change over time. One's perception of the life worth living is a function of numerous physical, historic, and social variables.[35] The potential for disagreement and debate about the identification and establishment of the good seems limitless. Each perception may contain elements that are and some that are not supported from a particular moral point of view. One might speculate that such a permissive atmosphere would result ultimately in a moral anarchy where each member functioned as a sovereign moral authority and concern for a common morality would perish. However, this is not the case. As demonstrated, there is a minimum common morality that binds particular moral communities and provides a moral identity to shared visions and commitments. A minimum common morality allows individuals to select, construct, and pursue their own version of the life worth living so long as such activity does not traverse the boundaries of the minimum common morality. Not only are individuals free to pursue their own ends, they are free to associate with others to pursue shared or mutually agreed-upon goals. Again, the subgroup is subject to the limitations or boundaries represented by the wider common morality. Thus, the importance of a wider common morality increases rather than decreases as individuality and plural perceptions of the good or the life worth living are tolerated and safeguarded.[36]

If notions of the good and life worth living, and the preferred means by which to achieve or approximate them, are individually, contextually, and dynamically held, it seems plausible to assume that no single end or state is sufficient to satisfy at once the requirements of such diversity. Thus, to hold an all-inclusive view of the good or goal of human life that is required and/or normative appears impossible in the modern West. If diversity is endorsed and protected, conflicts that turn on different notions of the life worth living are inevitable. It is also inevitable that moral agents will hold different views regarding the limit of one's duty to do to another his or her good. The principle of beneficence does not specify the extent to which one is morally obliged to risk one's own interests or good, or the interests and good of other persons, in order to fulfill one's duties to a particular individual. As with the identification of the good life, the cost sufficient to override a moral agent's duties of beneficence will be determined by one's particular moral commitments and an assessment of the particular circumstances that prompts a choice among goods or evils. More will be said in Chapters 6 and 7 about these matters. All that is intended for the present is to signal that particular moral communities and moral agents may hold diverse defensible views regarding the limits of a duty to do the good to another.

People who care for babies in neonatal nurseries may belong to a variety of moral communities and their respective identifications and rank orderings of goods and interests may differ. Parents may be Southern Baptist, the nurse a Reform Jew, the neonatologist an atheist, and the social worker a Roman Catholic. It is possible, even probable, that each party could reach a different reasonable decision, given their individual moral commitments, about what interventions ought to occur. Yet, only one party should have final say regarding the infant. The preceding discussion of the principle of self-determination, expressed in the context of neonatology as parental autonomy, proposed as a procedural premise that parents are the appropriate deciders except in certain instances. This conclusion, however, has not been universally accepted, as the discussion of possible alternate deciders in Chapter 4 will show. Nevertheless, settling the question of *who decides* only resolves one dilemma in neonatology. The decision about *what ought to be done* still remains.

Where a consensus regarding the care of certain impaired newborns is lacking, mutual respect for reasonable decisions necessarily is a cardinal feature. Without mutual respect, the prospect exists for the moral community to be plunged into conflict as particular communities seek to forcibly establish their vision of the good life. Mutual respect does not, however, require that a dissenter participate in an action judged to be a harm or wrong according to the dissenter's moral sense. The canon of mutual respect cannot support a duty to violate one's moral commitments. The principle of beneficence in the context of neonatology draws attention to the good or interest of the severely diseased or defective newborn. The good or interest of others, which may compete with the newborn, are drawn into the zone of decision making by the principle of justice.

Principle of Justice

Decisions for or against medical efforts to prolong the life of an imperiled newborn do not take place in a vacuum. Parents or others may attempt to discern the good or best interest of a neonate in isolation from other commitments. In actual practice, however, it is nearly impossible in these unfortunate situations to escape from considering the effect the neonate's continued life or early death may have on others, especially family members. It is not unusual, in my experience, for parents to perceive that their capacity to meet moral obligations to other children and/or vows to one another may be compromised or jeopardized by the requirements for care posed by the survival of a severely defective infant. The moral process of taking account of the legitimate claims of others in relation to the rights of or duties to a defective newborn falls within the realm of the principle of justice.[37] Simply stated, the principle of justice is concerned with the moral way in which benefits and burdens subject to human control ought to be imposed, shared, distributed, or allocated. Justice is done when one receives his or her due. An injustice occurs when benefits are denied or burdens imposed unduly.[38] The dilemma that parents face is that of determining what is rightfully due to competitors for their limited resources of love, nurture, and provision of opportunity, among other things, and why.[39] The answers that are variously given by parents reflect the diverse moral visions that they hold. In short, the effects of pluralism cannot be avoided even with issues of justice.

Theorists of justice tend to agree that equals ought to be treated equally and that unequals may be treated unequally. At issue, however, are the relevant properties or traits that qualify individuals or classes of individuals as equals or unequals.[40] The particular properties that make entities equal or unequal will reflect what a theorist has determined is valuable. This is to say that the determination of one's due (the substance of justice) is conceived; it is a human invention, not a human discovery or, necessarily, a revelation of absolutes from God (this, of course, depends on one's doctrine of revelation).[41] If this account is correct, then the dynamic character of rules of justice is partially explained. As values within a society change, the range of goods and services subject to principles of distributive justice is influenced. Similarly, as values within a society evolve, the relevant properties of individuals that determine standing within the moral community will be influenced. It should come as no surprise that some people conclude that certain classes of humans are unequal in relevant respects with other members of the moral community, such as to justify unequal claims to social resources. Thus, parents might conclude that it is morally proper to compare the interests of their children and determine that a preference for the claims of a healthy child over those of a severely defective neonate to familial resources is morally just. The judgments that particular parents reach, as indicated above, reflect their view of what establishes equal and unequal claims to certain resources.

More will be said about one's standing in moral communities, relative claims to benefits and against burdens, and balancing competing interests and duties in Chapter 4, where the environment of neonatology will be described, and in Chapter 5 where concepts of personhood will be reviewed. All that is desired now is to note the possibility for values, commitments, and duties to compete for priority when treatment decisions for defective newborns are required. The principle of justice is relevant to these situations of choice in the guidance it provides for the negotiation between conflicting interests and claims. Principles of justice are value-laden. They reflect particular orderings of value, commitment, and duty. The result in a moral pluralism is many orderings consistent with diverse moral visions. The principle of justice, while not specifying conduct for a particular situation, nevertheless, is useful as a general guide to conduct. It expands the scope of one's moral concern to include others with a material interest in the distribution of benefits and burdens that flow from a decision or action in a situation of scarcity. This suggests that in deciding the treatment or nontreatment of severely impaired newborns, parents and others may properly consider the benefit or burden their decision confers on others as well as on the neonate. The basic contribution of the principle of justice in these situations is that it requires parental choices between values, commitments, goals, and duties be based on morally relevant differences to justify any particular rationing of benefits and burdens.

In conclusion, this review of the principles of self-determination, beneficence, and justice began with an assertion that "hard cases" in neonatology may not submit to a single right decision for or against treatment of an imperiled newborn. Though these principles are believed relevant to moral dilemmas in neonatal medicine, what they are understood to mean and direct in particular cases will reflect value commitments of the decision maker and the moral community of which he or she is a member. This is only to state the obvious.

In an environment where certain and uniform answers to perplexing moral dilemmas are presently beyond reach, reasonable choices for particular cases merit respect. In such an environment, rational explanation and negotiation of diverse viewpoints is the only morally acceptable approach to the resolution of fundamental disagreements regarding what action is morally indicated in response to the birth of a defective newborn. Until differences are resolved and guidance is agreed upon by diverse moral communities, a sustained analysis of possible choices and their consequences will be a helpful means to choosing reasonably, if not rightly, in the eyes of all.

2

Parents and Children

Much of the discussion in medical ethics concentrates on determining the status of certain classes of patients and, as a result, what treatments or nontreatments are morally required on the basis of that status. Newborns, especially severely diseased or defective ones, are a class of patients about which there is disagreement concerning their standing in the moral community and the duties owed to them with respect to that standing. This uncertainty about what value to place on and what protections to extend to imperiled newborns is not new. As this chapter will show, understandings of the parent-child relation have evolved over time. Three features of these understandings are important to decisions regarding the fate of imperiled newborns. The first is that a primary objective for child-rearing practices has been the child's capacity to function independently in his or her own social system. The second is that parents generally have been held responsible to prepare their child for this independence. Third, parents have been accorded authority over their children commensurate with their duties. These features emerge when the parent-child relation is examined in history, philosophy, religion, and law. This record is important to the contemporary debate regarding the medical treatment of imperiled newborns to the extent that the precedents and perspectives derived from it address the questions of who is responsible for making decisions and what end should be advanced by these decisions.

Parent and Child in Historical, Philosophical, and Religious Perspective

It is a commonplace that practice influences theory and that theory influences practice. Regardless of the specific realm of activity, what is theoretically held about a practice and the ends it seeks will affect to a greater or lesser degree how that practice is pursued. The inverse is also true. How people actually undertake certain practices, conditioned by their time and place, influences to a greater or lesser degree what is theoretically held and how it is expressed conceptually. Thus it is reasonable to infer that philosophical and religious thought about the relationship between parent and child would and did affect popular beliefs about and expectations for the relationship, as well as the actual conduct of the parties.

Child-rearing is a practice that has been influenced by philosophical and theological conceptualizations and imperatives. The nature of the parent-child relationship, the respective duties and rights, and the norms of conduct for all not only have conditioned practice but practice has conditioned relevant philosophical and theological concepts, duties, rights, and norms. Here we survey the parent-child relation in history and in selected philosophical and religious literature. The individuals whose thoughts have been selected for review have variously influenced in important ways the development of Western secular and religious ideas regarding the parent-child relation, child-rearing practices, parental duties, and parental authority over children. As is the case with many histories of ideas, our review begins with Plato.

In his *Republic*, Plato (427?–347 B.C.) expressed his suspicions of the private family. He did not oppose the sentiments of family life. His worry was over the strength of those sentiments among the ruling class. For Plato, the guardians' primary loyalty should be the well-being of the ideal city. Loyalties within and to a private family or private property posed a threat to the performance of one's civic duty. As a consequence of this worry, Plato proposed that, due to their duties of oversight, children of the ruling class should be reared in a communal setting by members of the ruling class not involved in the administration of the city. He did not object to other classes, those ruled by their appetites, acquiring private property or being devoted to the family because by so doing their appetites were satisfied and the well-being of the

city would be served accordingly. But for the guardian the following law was proposed: "That these women [guardian women]
shall be common to all men, and that none shall cohabit with any
privately, and that the children shall be common, and that no
parent shall know its own offspring nor any child its parent."[1] In
the *Republic,* eugenic reproduction was favored, the best men and
best women cohabiting "in as many cases as possible and the
worst with the worst in the fewest, and that the offspring of the
one must be reared and that of the other not, if the flock is to be
as perfect as possible." How the inferior and those born defective
are to be eliminated, according to Plato, should be private to the
rulers in order to decrease dissension.[2] In a later work, *Laws,* Plato
observes that conceiving children is a serious matter. The partners
should be sober: "By consequence the drinker is an awkward,
bungling sower of his seed, and 'tis no wonder he commonly
begets shambling, shifty creatures with souls as twisted as their
bodies."[3]

The father in subject class families, according to Plato, had
great authority over his children. A child incurs a debt to parents
for his or her generation, care, and labor in his or her behalf during his or her youth. The debt of children, like the authority of
the father, is unequivocal. Under no circumstances can the honor
or authority of a parent be abridged, not even when a parent
threatens a child's life. In Plato's words, "In this sole case, when
a man's life is in danger from his parents, no law will permit slaying, not even in self-defense—the slaying of the father or mother
to whom his very being is due. The law's command will be that
he must endure the worst rather than commit such a crime."[4]

Aristotle (384–322 B.C.) parted company from Plato with regard to the need for communal care of children. Aristotle believed
that the family association was established by nature to provide
for everyday wants. Children are a common good to parents but
there are circumstances (deformity, overpopulation) in which certain children should be destroyed. In *Politics,* Aristotle writes: "As
to the exposure and rearing of children, let there be a law that no
deformed child shall live, but where there are too many (for in
our state population has a limit), when couples have children
in excess, and the state of feeling is averse to the exposure of
offspring, let abortion be procured before sense and life have begun. . . ."[5]

Children were important in Greek households. At least one

son and one daughter was considered desirable. The son would perpetuate the family and defend it on the battlefield and in the assembly. The daughter was a means by which parental aims could be realized through marriage. Children provided other securities, such as the continued worship of ancestors and the retention of all family property. Without a child heir, a man's property was absorbed by a close relative. As might be imagined in this environment, the Greek father had great power. Like Plato, Aristotle vested the father with supreme authority, likening him to a monarch whose rule is based on a more mature reason.[6] He rebuts Plato's preference for communal child-rearing as ineffective and impractical. The sort of unity or harmony envisaged by Plato would not be realized. Aristotle observes that people think primarily of their own interests and neglect those common duties that others can be expected to fulfill.[7]

The relationship between father and son (parent and child), according to Aristotle, is between unequals, as are husband and wife, ruler and subject. As author of a child's existense, the child "belongs" to the parents, and remains a part of the father's person until he or she becomes independent. "Friendship" or love should characterize the relationship between parent and child. It consists in giving, not receiving, affection, which is the proper virtue of friends. Paradoxically, Aristotle used mothers who give their children away to illustrate this claim. In his view, "It seems to be sufficient for them to see their children prosper and to feel affection for them, even if the children do not render their mother her due, because they do not know her."[8]

Parents incur in the process of generation obligations to maintain and educate their children. Love for children causes parents to fulfill these obligations, even if it requires a great sacrifice, like placing the child with others better able to provide for them. An aim for child-rearing is the child's self-sufficiency. A practice that viewed children (and wives) in common, like that articulated by Plato, would result in a weakened love that would undermine the performance of parental duties.

During the era of the Roman Empire, Cicero (106–43 B.C.) considered the home the foundation of civil government. The relationships of husband and wife and parent and child are two of several appropriate contexts for kindness. The degree of kindness to be shown to another, however, is in proportion to the closeness of the relationship. For example, the bonds of kinship were ranked below those of friendship and love of country but above those of citizenship in the same city-state and being of the same people, tribe, or tongue. Within the bond of kinship there also is a rank-ordering: "The first bond of union is that between husband and wife; the next, that between parents and children; then we find one home, with everything in common."[9] Cicero held that children are obligated to parents for the services the parents have provided. Parents, on the other hand, are obligated to "children and the whole family, who look to us alone for support and can have no other protection."[10] But he acknowledges that the performance of these duties can be tempered by circumstance. The parental application of duty or rule requires experience and practice, not unlike the way physicians and generals discharge their duty.[11]

The religious communities of Judaism and Christianity also consider parenting, child-rearing, and family areas of vital interest. But the scriptural picture of marriage, child-rearing, and parental authority tends to vary over time.[12] While the form of marriage moves from polygyny to an ideal of monogamy, the notion that children are a blessing or gift from God remains constant. So, too, the belief prevails that the father is God's representative, exercising an authority under God, responsible to God for the preparation of his children to be members of the covenant community (Deut. 4:9–10; 6:7, 21; 11:19; 31:12–13; Josh. 4:6–7; Ps. 78:4). The primary function of the wife and mother was to produce children. She had the responsibility of caring for them (Gen. 24:11, 13–16, 19–20; 27:9, 14; Matt. 33:33; 24:41; Titus 2:4–5) and could also exercise considerable authority over family life, second only to the father (Gen. 21:10; 27:11–17; Judg. 17:2–6).

Children were regarded as the property of the father during the early periods of biblical history. For example, they could be seized for debt (2 Kings 4:1) and daughters could be sold into marriage (Exod. 21:7–11). To acknowledge the authority of the father, however, is not to suggest that the parents were not to love their children (Gen. 22:2, 1 Kings 3:26). Children were perceived as a blessing from God (Ps. 127:1, 3; 128:3–4; Job 5:25), born into an idealized family characterized by beauty, strength, and affection (Gen. 22, 45; Ruth; 2 Sam. 18:33). Children were valued: Sons perpetuated the name and personality of the father (Gen. 38), and daughters were to marry, join her husband's family, and assume the responsibilities of motherhood. Sons and daughters were commanded by God to honor their father and mother (Exod. 20:12). They were cursed by God if they did not (Deut. 27:16). On the other hand, children without parents were seen as objects of special divine concern (Exod. 22:22-24). The importance of the family in Jewish life is evidenced by the use of the family as an image of relationship for all Israel and by its use among first-century Christians to refer to the Christian community.[13]

The official teaching of the Roman Catholic church regarding marriage, children, and the family has remained fairly constant through the centuries. Two personalities within Catholicism particularly have been important to an articulation and perpetuation of this teaching. The first is Saint Augustine (354–430), Bishop of Hippo, a dominant figure in his own time, and, through his writing, a major influence in the subsequent development of Roman Catholic thought. Consistent with biblical themes, Augustine taught that the power of parents is subordinated to the authority of God. Children are subjected by God to a kind of "free bondage" to their parents.[14] Children are seen as a blessing from God, and parents are obligated under God to nurture and educate them piously. The faithful performance of these duties warrants honor for the parents.[15]

St. Thomas Aquinas (1225–1274) tended to follow Aristotle more than Augustine about domestic matters. Aquinas believed that the good of children, not only their existence, is what nature intends by their birth. This means that parents must be concerned about more than just having a child. They must be concerned about the child's education and development until the child reaches maturity and the state of virtue. In agreement with Aristotle, Aquinas held parents responsible to provide three things for their children: existence, nourishment, and education. The end of child-rearing, he claimed, is self-sufficiency.[16] Aquinas believed that a child had status apart from the parents. He or she was an individual being with rights vis-à-vis the parents. The mother and father were obligated to provide for the physical, mental, moral, and religious education of a child in addition to the needs of domestic life. For this service, a child has duties of obedience and respect while young, and reverence throughout life.[17]

Many of the opinions of St. Augustine and St. Thomas are affirmed for contemporary Roman Catholics in a document, "Fos-

tering the Nobility of Marriage and the Family,'' issued by the
Second Vatican Council (1963–65), in which the family is presented as the ''foundation of society. In it the various generations
come together and help one another to grow wiser and to har-
monize personal rights with the other requirements of social life.''
The primary duty of parents is to lead children by example ''to
human maturity, salvation, and holiness. Graced with the dignity
and office of fatherhood and motherhood, parents will energeti-
cally acquit themselves of a duty which devolves primarily on
them, namely education, and especially religious education.''[18]

The theocentric perspective of Catholicism regarding marriage, family, and child-rearing is rooted in interpretations of
scripture and perpetuated through the teaching office of the
church. It is at the point of parental authority that these sources
move away from the earlier absolutism found in the oldest biblical
narratives. Augustine warned against applying biblical literalism
to morals. Aquinas held that children were individuals, bearers
of rights that merited respect. The Second Vatican Council speaks
of ''the surpassing ministry of safe-guarding life.'' It condemns
abortion and infanticide as ''unspeakable crimes.'' Positions such
as these surely limit the legitimate exercise of power by parents
over children.

Protestant reformers Martin Luther (1483–1546) and John Calvin (1509–64) deviated from the teaching of Catholicism regarding
marriage and family primarily by a displacement of celibacy in favor of the marital state as the ideal and norm. Their views on
domestic relations are similar.[19] They both taught that parental
authority is derived from God. Calvin believed that God set parents over children to teach them by example to fear the Lord.[20]
Luther called parents ''God's representatives'' in a position of
honor ''above all other persons on earth'' with a temporal and
spiritual authority over children.[21] The temporal authority is over
the necessities of and preparation for life; the spiritual authority
is to teach children the gospel.

Parental duties to beget and care for children were seen by
Luther as ''truly golden and noble works.'' He believed the no-
blest work of a woman is to bear children and that women were
to be comforted in childbirth by saying, ''Work with all of your
might to bring forth the child. Should it mean your death, then
depart happily, for you will die in a noble deed and in subser-
vience to God.''[22] Parents are due honor from children since it is

through parents that God gives children food, house and home, protection and security. Parents are trustees under God, responsible to "train and govern" children according to God's will. They are responsible under God to educate children for worldly success and to be concerned about their spiritual lives. The parental office, therefore, is "a strict commandment and injunction of God, who holds . . . [them] accountable to it."[23] Luther believed that parents could attain salvation or earn hell by the way they raised their children.[24]

Luther's attitudes toward physically deformed and mentally retarded beings were widespread in Europe from the Middle Ages to the Enlightenment. When asked for advice about a twelve-year-old backward child with a maliciously gleeful laugh, Luther recommended that the parents throw the child off a bridge into the water. They should be able to defeat a charge of homicide, counseled Luther, on the grounds that the child was merely a lump of flesh without a soul. He referred to malformed infants as changelings not created by God, but made by the devil. They either had no soul or the devil was their soul.[25]

The influence of this sort of superstition on the actual treatment of malformed infants is difficult to gauge. Similarly, it is difficult to know the extent to which the views of authorities from Plato to Calvin actually influenced valuations of children and child-rearing practices. It seems fair to conclude, however, from historical sources that the standing of all young children during this era was precarious.[26] Children, especially infants, in the ancient, medieval, and Renaissance worlds had a high risk for an early death at nature's or a human hand. Infant mortality was high and the emotional investment of parents in newborns prudentially was kept to a minimum.[27] Medicine was not very effective in the control of disease. Ancient pediatric doctrines were perpetuated. During the sixteenth and seventeenth centuries, in addition to changeling superstitions, it was believed that the status of a newborn was conditioned by the mother's behavior during pregnancy. For example, fright would result in a deformed infant, a rich diet would lead to the birth of a girl and a lean diet would produce a boy. Techniques of child care were basically matters of custom, often inattentive to many of the special needs of children.[28] Infanticide was tolerated despite increasing official civil and ecclesiastical protest. Infants that were female, deformed, born of an illicit union, or born to poor families particularly were in danger of being killed or abandoned without the mother or father incurring much risk of censure or punishment. Once born and not threatened by parental choice, infants were sent to "wet-nurse"[29] and were later "put out" (perhaps by age six or seven years) to an apprenticeship or some similar activity to learn of the adult world. The physical separation facilitated an emotional separation that provided a cushion if the child died at wet-nurse; a not uncommon event. Apprenticeships or similar placements for those children who survived infancy kept parents from becoming too attached to children who were still vulnerable. In addition, the children were prepared to take a place in society and their labors served an economic function. These practices of the "well-to-do" have been referred to as forms of "institutionalized abandonment."[30]

An attitude that children were not very important is evidenced during the fifteenth and sixteenth centuries in Europe, England, and colonial America. Restrained parental affection, care of infants by someone other than the mother, infanticide, abandonment, and deaths at wet-nurse all are reported. The lineal family was of greater importance than the nuclear family. Ties of blood had priority, for in them the honor of the line was transmitted, the integrity of inheritance was preserved, and the age and permanence of the family name was assured. The authority of the husband and father over wife and children was sanctioned by custom and law. Becoming attached to infants who might disappear would have been a premature investment of affection. Better to wait, to be somewhat detached, parents probably reasoned, than to establish an unlimited bond with a child whose survival was uncertain. For example, Cotton Mather, in colonial America, worried that his son Samuel would die in infancy. He wrote, "The convulsions of my own mind, were all this while, happily composed and quieted; and with much composure of mind, I often and often in prayer resigned the child unto the Lord."[31]

Besides being viewed with detachment by their parents, as well as being considered vulnerable, prior to the seventeenth century the precarious status of children was also characterized by almost total subjection to the power of the father. At least until the fifth century, arranged marriages and adoptions were means by which family property was acquired and perpetuated. Children could be used as political hostages, security for debts, or sold as slaves. A father's authority or power with regard to the care and nurture of his children was effectively maintained into the sixteenth century. The complaints of religious authorities and unenforced proscriptions in civil law were ineffective to alter certain paternal prerogatives or parental practices sanctioned by social custom, e.g., infanticide. State protection of children was almost completely limited to the destitute or abandoned. Paternal power was protested when it was perceived as unduly harsh but little else was done.

William Blackstone's commentaries on the English Common Law discuss parental duties to legitimate children and parental power over them. Parents were obligated for the maintenance, protection, and education of their children. The maintenance required was limited to those "necessaries" to life.[32] With regard to protection, there was a legal indulgence of the aggressions of a father against another in defense of his child. And finally, the duty to educate was considered of greater importance than any. Blackstone approvingly quotes Puffendorf: "It is not easy to imagine or allow, that a parent has conferred any considerable benefit upon his child, by bringing him into the world; if he afterwards entirely neglects his culture and education, and suffers him to grow up like a mere beast, to lead a life useless to others, and shameful to himself."[33]

The power of parents was based on their duties to maintain, protect, and educate their children. Such power was necessary to perform these duties and was "partly . . . a recompence for his care and trouble in the faithful discharge of it."[34] Parents, among other things, were empowered by English law to correct, promote obedience, consent to the marriage of a minor child (majority was reached at the age of twenty-one years even though certain rights were attained by boys at age twelve and by girls at age seven), retain the income from a son's estate during his minority, and benefit from the child's labor while supported by the father. A mother, as such, was entitled to reverence and respect, but not power equal to a father's.

Early American legal doctrines regarding the power of parents and the status of children drew upon this British background. If the parental obligations of maintenance or education were not met and it fell upon the colony to do so, the colony could legally order a child to work or into an apprenticeship in order that its support would not burden the community. According to the Act of 1641 of the Colony of New Plymouth, it would be lawful under these circumstances for the township "to take order that those children bee put to worke in fitting Imployment according to theire strength and abillitie or placed out by the townes."[35] In those instances in which parents willfully or by circumstance did not meet their obligations to children, the community, at least in colonial America, assumed the parental power that had been forfeited. Like chattel, a child was held by others and only minimally recognized by custom or law to have interests of his or her own.

The general picture of children as vulnerable to nature's whims and human judgments, detached physically and emotionally from parents and kin, and subject to an almost unrestrained paternal power suggests that, in the main, children lived on the edge of family and social life prior to the seventeenth century. They enjoyed a limited status and endured a precarious existence. Though there were exceptions to the general description provided here, and even though signs of change are apparent earlier, children did not emerge in a major way as a focal point of family life until around the seventeenth century. Profound changes were set in motion that have led to contemporary views of children, families, and child-rearing that are radically inconsonant with the past.

Social historian Philippe Aries considers the seventeenth century pivotal in the history of children. This century in Europe marks a time in which the special needs of children began to be recognized. This recognition basically coincided with the development of the concept of the family in conjugal rather than lineal terms. There was a turn inward that resulted in the movement of children from a precarious to a protected status. Prior to this time, Western society in general gave little attention to the particularity of childhood—it was the period in which a child could not care for himself or herself. Between the ages of six and nine, the child moved into the adult world, into a larger group in which learning took place by helping adults do what they do. But toward the end of the seventeenth century, apprenticeship declined and formal education began to rise. Children learned about life in schools, not in the world. Parental affection came to be seen as more obligatory with the encouragement of the Catholic Church, Protestant Reformers, and the state. Families began to organize around children, whose length of stay in the home increased because of changing educational practices and a declining infant

mortality. The lineal family and the community retreated as pri-
·mary contexts of sociability. The home became the center of private social contact. The conjugal family became valued in itself
and as a secure context for emotion.

The growing influence of Christianity contributed to these
changing perceptions and practices. The social implications of
Christian teaching that children had immortal souls, just like
adults, seemed finally to affect family life and child-rearing practices. The notion that childhood was a time of innocence gained
credibility, despite the belief that children were conceived in sin.
Religious emphases not only began to influence the common person, they also began to be used by philosophers as additional
warrants for their ideas. Religious doctrines together with cultural
and social changes between 1500 and 1700 provided considerable
ferment for developing conceptualizations of children and domestic relations.

Thomas Hobbes (1588–1679) thought that children should be
in absolute subjection to the one who nurtures and preserves.
Preservation as the key to legitimate dominion is indicated by a
comment on exposure and abandonment, ''and if the mother shall
think fit to abandon, or expose her child to death, whatsoever
man or woman shall find the child so exposed, shall have the
same right which the mother had before; and for this reason,
namely, for the power not of generating, but preserving.''[36] But
even though subject to and obedient to parents, children, by an
indulgence of the parents, are considered ''free-men.''[37]

In a later work, *Leviathan*, Hobbes finds the basis of paternal
power in a child's expressed or implied consent evidenced by his
or her obedience to the parents.[38] This basis also suggests that
Hobbes did not consider children the property of their parents.
The consent grants permission for parents to rule. The state can
impose upon parents obligations to care for and support children.
If they fail to do so the state can intervene to protect children.
The state, therefore, can lessen the danger of injury to each at the
hands of another. Gratitude, in a political society, becomes the
ground for obedience to parents, not fear for one's life.[39]

Hobbes frequently cites biblical texts to support his views.
John Locke (1632–1704) similarly employed biblical texts and religious precepts to buttress his arguments concerning the status
of children and the nature of parental authority. Locke reasoned
that parental authority is natural. No civil law can set a father's

power over a mother's since, according to God, both are to be honored.[40] He observes that parental rule is temporary. Age and reason free children from subjection to parents. They are not born in a state of equality with adults but they are born to it, i.e., they mature or grow into it. Parental powers, therefore, are limited by and directed to the good of a child. Parents are to care for children "during the imperfect state of childhood. To inform the mind and govern the actions . . . til reason shall take its place and ease them of that trouble. . . . "[41] Until a child is freed by reason, a parent has a right and duty to understand and will for a child. "Lunatics and idiots," for example, who never develop reason, are never freed from the government of their parents.[42] Thus, Locke believed that parental power stems from an acceptance of the responsibility to provide for the child's growth and development into a reasoning person. The family exists to serve the child, the child does not exist to serve the family. God instills by nature, according to Locke, a desire and duty within parents to beget, nourish, and educate a child for freedom or independence.[43] Accordingly, Locke's theory of parenthood emphasizes parental duties rather than parental rights.

Whereas Locke focused on the development of reason as an end of parental action, Jean-Jacques Rousseau (1712–78) called attention to the place of feeling in and the process of the development of children. In *Emile*, Rousseau criticizes the child-rearing practices that separated the child from his or her mother, father, and home. He believed that children had special needs that could be satisfied better by parental care in the home. Mothers should nurse; fathers should educate.[44]

Rousseau's interest in the development, rather than the control, of children was shared by Jeremy Bentham (1748–1832) but expressed differently. Bentham favored keeping children under the immediate authority of parents rather than under the authority of laws that cannot adapt as readily during the process of growing up. Infants were seen as "feeble," "imperfect" beings who required continual protection until their physical and intellectual powers matured. Bentham considered mothers and fathers to be best suited to bear the responsibilities of nurture and education because they have the greatest facility to do so and because "natural affection disposes them to this duty. . . . "[45] Henry Sidgwick (1838–1900) also based his understanding of the duties of parent and child on the natural affection between them. Children were considered natural objects of compassion by parents because of the children's helplessness. Parents, "with tender and watchful care," according to Sidgwick, ought to promote their child's happiness but not without limit. Indicative of his utilitarianism, Sidgwick, wrote: "It seems unreasonable that he [parent] should purchase a small increase of their happiness by a great sacrifice of his own; and moreover there are other worthy and noble ends which may (and do) come into competition with it."[46] The family was considered the institution within which obligations to children could be met. In return, children owe gratitude to their parents. But existence alone is not considered a sufficient reason for gratitude. Sidgwick writes, "It may be said that a child owes gratitude to the authors of its existence. But life alone, apart from any provision for making life happy, seems a boon of doubtful value, and one that scarcely excites gratitude when it was not conferred from any regard for the recipient."[47]

In Europe, England, and America, the seventeenth century roughly marks the initiation of familial and social changes that would have a profound impact on the status of children. Family life reorganized to protect children and to provide for their needs. Programs to provide for children whose parents were unable or unwilling to do so became public commitments. Affection was no longer a superficial sentiment for parents. On the contrary, parental affection became seen as a providential implant, endorsed by civil law, to motivate parents to maintain, protect, and educate their children. The length of childhood increased as formal education replaced apprenticeships as the means by which children were prepared for an independent existence in the adult world. The impotency, despair, and fatedness of parents, suggested by the attitudes and child-rearing practices in some societies and during certain periods prior to the seventeenth century, gave way to a more universal hope for the future. Children became special, important, and valued by family and society alike. What is learned from the history of childhood is in reality a lesson about adulthood and parenthood, for in the story of child care through the centuries we do not find an evolution occasioned by children themselves. Rather, we find an evolving recognition by parents and other adults of a special status for children, their special needs, and a greater ability to satisfy needs that begin in infancy and evolve until the child attains maturity or independence.

Two major developments bear on the focus of this volume.

The first is a movement to see the family as a cornerstone and paradigm of social life. The second is a movement to see children as having interests both as a part of and apart from their parents and family. On the basis of these perceptions, parental authority can be conceived of in terms of a trust grounded in duties toward children. If this is correct, and I believe that it is, then a model for contemporary parent-child relations in normal circumstances would properly include three key features. First parental authority over children should be exercised in ways that foster a child's independence as defined in social and familial terms. The trust that parents hold is for the primary benefit of their child, sanctioned by reason, nature, or God, and enforced by law. The authority of parents becomes limited to the period in which a child is dependent upon parents, understood broadly as their minority and immaturity. Second, parental affection is a stimulus for the proper performance of parental duties and a safeguard against an abusive exercise of parental authority. Parental rights are limited to that which is necessary to fulfill parental duties, understood broadly as nurture and education. Third, mother and father have equivalent status, power, authority, and responsibility in relation to children. The beliefs and customs that sanctioned the superiority of men and the rule of fathers have yielded to egalitarian impulses. Women are now valued for purposes other than their childbearing and child-rearing gifts.

This understanding of the parent-child relation appears to accurately capture the main lineaments of the histories of thought and practice accepted by contemporary culture. It informs the tasks of making treatment decisions for imperiled newborns in several ways. First, it constitutes a strong endorsement for the presumption that parents are in authority and responsible to make these decisions. Second, it presents the child's independence or self-sufficiency as a primary objective of parental decisions and conduct. Third, it limits parental power to that which is commensurate with their duties. Fourth, it respects the integrity of the family and invests value in each of its members. In short, this analysis helps to answer the questions associated with the medical treatment of imperiled newborns: Who decides? What end should be sought?

Philosophers and theologians necessarily rely on the powers of persuasion and the force of reason to establish a concept, norm, or conduct. Law, on the other hand, is supported by the power of the state in establishing norms of conduct on the basis of legal concepts and principles. Moral theory, either of the philosophical or theological variety, may define what people ought to do but the law, in the usual course of events, defines what people may or must do. The principles and rules of American law have been applied to the parent-child relationship. It is to this aspect of our consideration of the status of children that we now turn.

A Delicate Balance: Parent and Child in Law

The law is a means by which the state expresses its interests. The relation between parent and child is one in which the state's interest has been stated rather ambivalently. On the one hand, the state has valued the integrity of the family and has resisted interfering in the relation between parent and child. On the other hand, the state has taken notice of the imbalance of power between parent and child and has sought to protect children when considered necessary. Balancing the interests of children, parents, and state is not an easy task for the law to perform. Statutes are usually too rigid to accommodate the unique circumstances of individual cases of conflict. Case law may not articulate a consistent legal standard since it is subject to the prejudices of individual judges. Yet despite these difficulties in application, the law contains standards and principles by which domestic relations are governed.

From a legal point of view, the status of children as bearers of rights normally begins at birth. This does not mean, however, that the law ignores the infant's or child's dependency. Because of this dependency or inability to exercise rights, the law follows nature and custom in recognizing parents as the primary representatives of a child's interests. Some legal experts suggest that parents do not have an independent right to make decisions for a child. They do so as a substitute for an incapable "person." Parents are placed in this substitutionary role by statute and judicial opinion because they are seen, rightly or wrongly, to know best their child's *existing* views and the value preferences of the family unit, which are seen to be a major contributor to the child's *future* views.[48] The legal relation of parent and child respects the natural relation created by conception and birth. As a result, parents are seen as the natural guardians of a child within a family that is considered a self-governing entity under the parents' discipline.[49]

The law presumes that an adult parent has "the capacity, authority and responsibility to determine and to do what is good for one's children." [50] This presumption of interest and capacity extends from the decision to conceive children[51] to decisions that determine a child's upbringing. Courts have protected parental authority with respect to child-rearing,[52] education,[53] and religious training.[54] Generally speaking, parents have a right and a duty to make decisions on behalf of their child, within reasonable limits, free from external interference.[55]

Parental duties, like parental rights, are defined only generally in the law. The enforcement of these duties is left mainly to moral sanction. It would be impossible for the state to inquire in every instance if and how parents have fulfilled their duties. Thus the law presumes that parents will protect the interests of a child who is also presumed in the law to have distinct and independent interests from those of the parents. This presumption of separable interests is subject to challenge.[56] It implies that a child is an autonomous individual rather than an individual developing autonomy. A young child is a dependent being, clearly not able to know or advance his or her own interests. Further, it is difficult to see how a young child's interests can be determined apart from the interests of those individuals with whom his or her destiny is linked in a material way. The notion that a child's interests can be determined apart from a consideration of his or her environment and relationships is questionable at best. Humans are social beings. Our self-perceptions are partly conditioned by our experience with other humans. Our roles in life are defined by our relationships with others. Our ability to realize certain potentials is dependent to greater and lesser degrees on the cooperation, benevolence, and respect of others. If interests are related to self-concepts, roles, and opportunities, as I think they partially are, then to imagine that a child's interests can be determined independently of relationships that in reality condition his or her interest is to misperceive the nature of the human condition. Holding such a view would entail a distortion of reality. Accordingly, it is more realistic to define a healthy or ill child's interests in relation to those persons and factors that, in fact and in important ways, define what his or her interests actually are. The relevant context and persons for determining an imperiled infant's interests are, in my opinion, its family.

State protection of the privacy and autonomy of the family seems based on the view that such protection is in the interest of the well-being of children. "Children are seen as dependent and in need of direct, intimate and continous care by the adults who are personally commited to assume such responsibility."[57] Biological parents are usually assigned to this task. If the natural relationship fails, however, the state assigns the parental relationship and associated duties to other willing adults. "Responsibility for the child, for his survival, for his physical and mental growth, for his eventual adaptation to community standards, thus becomes that of the designated adults in a family to whom the child, in his turn, is responsive and accountable."[58]

The law normally protects the integrity of the family. A statement by a New York judge is representative of the reverence with which the family is held in the law: "[t]he filial bond is one of the strongest, yet most delicate, and most inviolable of all relationships."[59] This sort of support assumes the competency of families. As legal scholar Joseph Goldstein and colleagues note, the law "neither has the sensitivity nor the resources to maintain or supervise the on-going day-to-day happenings between parent and child—and these are essential to meeting ever-changing demands and needs. Nor does it have the capacity to predict future events and needs, which would justify or make workable over the long run any specific conditions it might impose concerning, for example, education, visitation, health care, or religious upbringing."[60] In addition, legal sanction of parental duties helps to keep the support of children from becoming a public burden.[61]

Rights of privacy undergird the family as a context for intimacy and sharing. Laurence H. Tribe, professor of law at Harvard University, observes that the first amendment has been the basis upon which courts have protected the integrity and vitality of human associations, including the family. In a comment on *Griswold v. Connecticut*, the U.S. Supreme Court decision barring state prohibition of contraception within marriage, Tribe suggests that a right to self-definition implicit in this decision is "incompatible with conferring upon any outsider a decisional role . . . "[62] regarding the size or constitution of a family.

The law, then, sanctions parental authority to the degree that it is necessary to fulfill parental duties to a child and the state. The duties are broadly understood to include maintenance ("necessaries" such as suitable shelter, food, and clothing),[63] education, medical care, and moral/religious training to a degree sufficient for a child's independent social existence. The state tends to be reluctant to interfere with family privacy and parental autonomy in the performance of these duties. The law does not penalize parents for failure to perform duties that are beyond their means or for omissions when a danger was not known to exist. Also, there is no violation of duty when there is no law supporting one side of a reasonable disagreement about how to fulfill parental duties. Similarly, parents are excused when they reasonably believe that they are serving the child's interest.[64]

The state reserves the right to intervene in the parent-child relation when such intervention is believed necessary to protect a child's or its own interest. State intervention in family matters rests on its police power and its *parens patriae* power. The police power is invoked "both to prevent . . . citizens from harming one another and to promote all aspects of the public welfare." For example, police power would be involved in the prevention of child abuse. The *parens patriae* power is "the state's limited paternalistic power to protect or promote the welfare of certain individuals, like young children and mental incompetents, who lack the capacity to act in their own best interests."[65] Legislation prescribing vaccination, establishing compulsory education, and regulating the conditions of work are expressions of the state's *parens patriae* power. The state's own interests and the interests of children in general are seen to be served by these requirements. Parental judgments about other matters are presumed competent and not subject to state intervention unless it is shown that the parents are either unfit, unable, or unwilling to care for a child adequately.

Some of the state's exercise of its *parens patriae* power has been criticized. Critics charge that it has been used to uphold standards of child neglect that are broad and subject to ad hoc analysis by social workers and judges. These decisions may reflect personal values regarding child-rearing rather than demonstrable evidence of present or probable harm to a child.[66] "After all," says legal scholar Stuart Baskin, "at the heart of most child-welfare decisions is essentially a value judgment as to 'what kind of a child one hopes to produce.' Substituting the state's decision for the parents' often simply means accepting a judge's child-rearing judgments over those of the parents. Yet, the values of . . . judges, like those of others, are reflections of their personal biases and— more importantly in a society where judges are drawn from the middle class while state intervention is often against poor families—of their class biases."[67]

To counteract a misapplication of the *parens patriae* power in neglect proceedings, critics urge that the court's interests be restricted to the *process* of parental decision making. Alexander Capron, a lawyer, writes, "[P]arental authority should be superseded only if the judge has been convinced by clear and convincing proof that the parents, through lack of attention, incapacity, or adverse interest, are unable to represent their child's interests." Further, "restricting judicial oversight to whether parents are 'fully informed and acting in good faith' for a particular child rather than the acceptability of the decision is also less intrusive on the interests in familial privacy and continuity of care that are important parts of our jurisprudence. . . . "[68] These several objections to *parens patriae* are sufficient to indicate some of the problems associated with its use. Accordingly, the state should only reluctantly and as a last resort invoke this power in regard to the medical care of severely diseased or defective newborn infants. These are situations bursting with value-based disagreements regarding an infant's interests. The good for the child or its best interests may be subject to more than one valid interpretation. When this is the case, and in view of the state's respect for family privacy, the state properly should defer to the informed and reasonable judgments of those persons (parents and medical personnel) intimately involved.

This brief review suggests that the law is hesitant to interfere in the relation of parent and child. The law tends to uphold the view that parents, in the language of the U.S. Supreme Court, "have the right, coupled with the high duty, to recognize and prepare [their children] for additional obligations."[69] Parents are presumed to have the capacity, maturity, and experience that children lack to make decisions. And because of the natural bonds of affection, parents usually can be trusted to act in the best interests of their children. The same Court observed that a failure to do this "is hardly a reason to discard wholesale those pages of human experience that teach that parents generally do act in the child's best interests. . . . The statist notion that governmental power should supersede parental authority in *all* cases because *some* parents abuse and neglect children is repugnant to American tradition.''[70] The state can rely on its police power and *parens patriae* power to intercede in those cases where parents, for whatever reason, do not conform to the presumptions of the law.

A Concluding Proposition

Children in history and from the perspectives of philosophy, religion, and law have been considered mainly in relation to their parents. This is especially true for infants and young children whose dependency on parents is most direct. A perception that parents are disposed and equipped to manage a child during his or her period of dependency has led to a strong presumption that parents are responsible for the care and nurture of their children. This responsibility has been seen to carry with it a commensurate authority or power sufficient to perform those duties usually assigned to parents. A primary duty of parents can be expressed as a goal or objective for child-rearing. It is explicit or implicit in the thoughts of Plato, Aristotle, ancient Jewish writers, St. Thomas, Luther, Calvin, Locke, Rousseau, Sidgwick, English and American law, and discernible in practice. In short, parents are to direct their activities toward the production of a being whose life is useful to him or her and to others. I shall refer to this duty and goal as the development of a child's capacities for independence. Except in those instances in which parents judged an infant's death preferable to continued existence, for whatever reasons or to serve whatever interests, parents or parental surrogates have been considered responsible for nurturing a child and preparing it to be self-determining in the moral sense of the term.

That a child's independence or self-sufficiency has been considered a primary end toward which parental activity should be directed seems indisputable. Though the language and means by which it has been expressed have changed over time, the goal seems to have been considered reasonable and worthy almost universally in custom, morality, and law. Its reasonableness and worthiness may explain why it has endured. It also may have endured because the capacities sufficient for independence are not specified. It does not establish a uniform method by which it is attained. Neither does it exclude a retention of some measure of voluntary dependency between parent and child, between members of an extended family, or between unrelated persons.

The notion that a child's independence is a worthy and primary objective for reproduction and child-rearing is as valid today as it was perceived to be by past generations. It reflects what usually is taken to be a natural part of the life cycle and human association. This is to say that independence fits comfortably with the view that parenting involves more than giving life to a new human being. According to this argument, children ought to be raised to be capable of making choices, including choices to leave parents and establish relationships apart from those based on kinship. In addition, certain goods are associated with a child's independence. Parents are liberated from the constraints of child care to pursue other goods. Children are freed to formulate life-plans, adopt values, pursue goals, and establish identities that are their own. Society has a chance to gain a productive member. And finally, as the cycle is repeated, a family and nation are perpetuated. Too many nonproductive, dependent members could threaten the existence of either a family or nation with limited resources. In short, the goal of independence and parental oversight was and is valid for several reasons: (1) It promotes certain esteemed goods and values. (2) Parents are usually effective in directing the process toward independence. (3) Parental responsibility for children is an efficient means by which to achieve this primary objective, except in unusual circumstances where parents disqualify themselves for the task. (4) Discrediting independence as a primary goal and/or displacing parents as primarily responsible for its realization, where possible, would constitute a significant deviation from our cultural past and would alter the character of the family and society in significant ways.

It is difficult to stipulate what capacities are necessary for independence. One can imagine that the criteria in a primitive culture would be radically different from that in contemporary urban society. The capability to hunt and kill game surely was important and perhaps necessary to one's existence in the distant past. These skills are not so important or necessary today for a computer analyst living in a city. This simple contrast suggests that criteria of independence are created, not discovered. They are relative to time, place, and social commitments. For example, independence may be attainable for a person with no legs in a society where wheelchairs are provided and the necessities of life are available on a market or welfare basis. It may not be attainable in a society organized differently.

There may be no universal, objective criteria for independence. Rather, the end of independence for children may express a universal value preference. Its formulation at any particular time and place can take account of resources and commitments that can minimize impairments that otherwise might negate the prospect for independence. This means that the path to independence is historically, culturally, scientifically, physically, economically, and in other ways conditioned. As a formal objective, independence does not dictate what capacities or values are sufficient to attain it. But perhaps more importantly for this inquiry, it allows for individualized approaches to children, some with unique abilities and talents, others with unique handicaps and incapacities. Parents are expected, according to this view, to take account of the particular circumstances of a child within the family and social contexts, and to adapt their goal-directed behaviors and considered judgments accordingly. With these qualifications in mind, a child's *minimal* independence toward which parental activity should be directed would include a capability to relate, communicate, ambulate, and perform tasks of basic hygiene, feeding, and dressing.[71] Clearly there are technologies available today that can supplement or compensate for one's deficiencies in any of these areas. If competent medical opinion is that a particular newborn is physically and/or mentally impaired to the degree that these capabilities are not attainable even with technological assistance, then parents and society are not obliged to attempt the impossible. Either or both may elect to sustain this class of newborns, but there can be no moral obligation to do the impossible. This conclusion obviously rests on the belief that independence and these criteria for minimal independence are morally defensible ends upon which duties to attain them are grounded.

Independence is a goal that, in reality, only can be approximated. "No man is an island," so the saying goes. Self-sufficiency is a notion that either ignores or denies the fact that people tend to require others to satisfy a range of needs and desires that are, at least as far as we know, distinctively human, e.g., to be loved. These qualifications suggest that independence as a basic goal in child-rearing cannot be pressed too far and still retain its viability. The capability for independence that is sought for children by parents ought, therefore, to be properly understood in minimal and culturally dependent terms. The standard for independence may be exceeded, potentially conferring upon the child additional opportunities, and potentially conferring upon others additional benefits. But when independence is not attainable, neither parents nor others are morally obliged, according to this argument, to provide for the dependent being's support. Parental decisions to prolong or not to prolong the life of a newborn infant reasonably believed never able to attain a minimal independence ought not to be qualified by law, policy, or any other authority. If society rejects the standard of minimal independence and mandates that parents sustain a perpetually dependent being, then society incurs an obligation to supplement parental resources to the extent necessary for these mandated obligations to be fulfilled. Without this commitment, the moral justification for societally enforced support is weakened. Absent this commitment, reasonable parental decisions that take account of an infant's condition within its familial and societal contexts ought to be respected.

3

Critically Ill Newborns: Parental Responses and Responsibilities

T HE HISTORICAL OVERVIEW provided in the preceding chapter indicated that an individual in the role of parent, either by reproduction or adoption, incurs obligations toward children and, perhaps, society. The performance of obligations, inherent to the parental role, to preserve and educate a child aims at the transformation of a child from a position of absolute dependence to an independence within a social order characterized by the interdependence of relatively independent persons. Custom, morality, and law have tended to affirm this objective for parenting without necessarily standardizing the means by which it was to be attained. Parents have been given broad discretionary authority to effect this end in the manner that they considered appropriate and within the limits of their means. The relationship between parent and child has been seen as an intimate one, grounded in affection, and inviolable except in extreme circumstances. The extent of parental authority or power over a child has been proportionate to their duties. As a child becomes more able to provide the necessities of life the responsibility, and therefore authority, of the parent decreases accordingly. Eventually, the parent and child stand as equals, in the vast majority of instances, even though the role-relation of parent and child persists.

Social and legal protection of this sort of parent-child relation has been based on the judgment that, in the main, it best serves a child's and society's interests. Primarily only in extreme circumstances have interferences by others been sanctioned. These instances usually involve a parental judgment or action that represents an injustice or unreasonable threat, all things considered, to a child who is considered incompetent to know, protect, or advance his or her own interests. When protective interventions fail some children are injured or harmed. The moral community expresses its condemnation of these injustices by ostracizing or penalizing the offender in some way. Though particular cases of parental failure may be invidious, they have not been seen sufficient to disrupt a long tradition of respect for parental authority and freedom to manage their children. In this chapter I propose a model of parenting in which parents have a quasi-fiduciary role and authority with respect to the care of children. It is argued that some measure of control and freedom to act is required in order to respond appropriately to the unpredictable risks or threats to children or family that may arise. Further, the parental autonomy advocated here is believed to be appropriate to contemporary patterns of family formation, which seem to aim at enhancing the quality of family life. In the process of developing this model of parenting, we shall take note of several phenomena and their implications for parental responses to the birth of a premature, low birth weight, or otherwise defective infant.

The Family in Transition

There can be no doubt that the family continues to change. The notion that children would mature, complete their education, marry, start a career and a family, never divorce, live in one place throughout life, and derive pleasure from seeing the cycle repeated through their own offspring has fallen on hard times. Marriages are being postponed, fewer children are desired, divorce is common, and family roles are changing.

The time between marriage and the birth of the first child is increasing. The median interval between the first marriage and the first child was fifteen months in 1960. By the late 1970s, the median interval was over two years. By the third year of marriage only 20 percent of couples were still childless in the early 1960s whereas by the end of the 1970s this number more than doubled to over 40 percent. This deemphasis on childbearing is also seen in the number of children that couples desire. The number of births expected or desired by wives between the ages of eighteen and thirty-four fell from 3.1 in 1965 to 2.3 in 1978. For those wives between eighteen and twenty-four in 1978 the average was 2.1, or roughly at the zero-population-growth level.[1]

Another indication of changing attitudes toward parenting is the use of contraception. The rate of contraception use by married women fluctuated within a narrow range between 1965 and 1976 (a low, in 1965, of 64.1 percent; a high, in 1973, of 70.5 percent).[2] These data clearly suggest that a significant number of wives wish to determine the number of children they bear and when to do so. The increase in legal abortions since 1973 underscores this point. There were approximately 745,000 legal abortions in the year in which the U.S. Supreme Court struck down statutes making abortion a crime. By 1984, the number of legal abortions was approximately 1.5 million.[3] Fertility and birth rates are decreasing. The fertility rate (basically the number of births that an average woman would have in her lifetime) has decreased from 2.9 in 1965 to 1.8 in 1979, less than the 2.1 zero-population-growth level. Birth rates also are declining. In 1965, there were 96.6 live births per 1,000 women fifteen to forty-four years of age. By 1979, the number of live births dropped almost 30 percent to 68.5 per 1,000 women in this age category.[4]

The size of families has also declined. The average family size in 1965 was 3.7 persons. By 1981, the average was 3.25.[5] The reduced size may be due to a decrease in the number of children or it may reflect a rise in the number of single-parent families. By the end of the 1970s, one in seven families in the United States was headed by a divorced, separated, widowed, or never-married woman. Regardless of the explanation, family size is clearly growing smaller. Between 1965 and 1981, the number of families with no or one child increased from 61.1 percent to 69.3 percent. Further evidence of a preference for fewer children is seen in the declining number of families with three or more children (22.1 percent in 1965, 10.9 percent in 1982).[6]

Smaller families have an effect on the quality of family life. A study by the University of Michigan Survey Research Center, completed in 1972, attempted to determine the impact that the number of children has on the quality of family life. Over 5,000 families were followed for five years. The study found that women with fewer children were more likely to enter the labor force, increasing their family incomes. A larger income divided by fewer family members results in a greater possible per capita expenditure. The educational attainment of children in the sample was found to be related to parental income and family size. The larger the family income and the smaller the family, the higher the educational achievement of the children. Two-wage-earner families tended to have fewer children than one-wage-earner families. Increasing family income and limiting family size in order to enhance the quality of life and opportunity of each child seems to take into account the dollar cost of raising children. Estimates vary, but for a middle-income family, the cost of raising a child from birth through four years at a state university is at least $100,000 in 1980 prices.[7]

The changing patterns of reproduction and family structure surveyed here suggest a movement in this country toward fewer children with births coming later in life. This trend appears encouraged by the advancement of women in education and careers, and by a changing social consciousness, effective contraception, and abortion. An effect of these transitions is an apparent heightened concern for the quality of family life, including the quality of children's lives.

Parenting: A Risky Venture

A tendency toward fewer and planned pregnancies would seemingly elevate the expectations that attend each pregnancy. Being pregnant is less and less considered the situation of the woman alone. Couples routinely report that "they" are pregnant. Describing pregnancy in this way implies that it is a cooperative venture that involves each partner in the hope, anticipation, and preparation for birth. Couples become pregnant and desire children for a variety of reasons, some admirable and others seemingly less worthy.

Some pregnancies are accidental. Contraception may fail, or perhaps the risk of pregnancy was not acknowledged. Abortion is one way to deal with an accidental or unwanted pregnancy. Obviously, these pregnancies were not desired. Another way to respond to an accidental pregnancy is to bring it to term. Twelve percent of all births in 1976 were reported as unwanted by the mothers.[8]

Jeffrey Blustein, a philosopher, observes that reasons for wanting children are many, and vary between cultures and historical periods. Some people may desire children in order to promote social goals apart from or in addition to the goals of the reproductive unit itself. Children also can serve economic interests as labor, income sources for a family, or financial or other support in old age. Some parents may be concerned with extending the blood line or family name. Some may wish to have someone to dominate or to use as a means to exhibit competence in a social role. Others may see children as a way to some form of immortality or an indispensable developmental milestone. Still others may see parenthood as a way of fulfilling the wishes or expectations of others, especially one's own parents. And finally, probably a high percentage of couples simply "want children for the altruistic pleasure of having them, caring for them, helping them grow and develop."[9]

Pregnant couples tend to imagine their future child as an object of their love, commitment, and sacrifice. Partners who become parents are usually motivated to extend their resources for the care and development of children with the expectation that the process and result will carry within it its own reward. They may dream of the child's achievement, beauty, intelligence, wit, charm, grace, or character.[10] They may speculate about the baby's sex, coloring, and which features of mom and dad the baby will have. Engaging in these fantasies and speculating about the bright future for this son or daughter can fill many hours during the long, nine-month waiting period. The child's first experiences may be imagined with pride and pleasure: his or her first word, step, day at school, religious communion, visit with grandparents, date, group activity, or pet. The list of possible events is endless. Names are considered, clothing and infant care products are purchased, the home is rearranged to receive the baby, parties may be held that involve others in the pregnancy, and attachments to the in utero infant begin. The anticipatory thrill associated with these activities, dreams, hopes, and fantasies may obscure any possibility of future problems, difficulties, hardships, disappointments, or failures. There may be an awareness of the potential risks and pitfalls of parenting, but they may not be expressed in a way that materially connects the risk with the current pregnancy. It is frightening for parents to think that this pregnancy might result in the birth of an infant with a serious impairment that could effectively shatter all the hopes and dreams they have for this child.

The contingent nature of life and health, though known to all, are effectively denied in daily life. There is no better symbol of hope than a child. People of goodwill, benevolently disposed to children tend not to reproduce when the future looks grim or catastrophic. Placing an innocent individual in a situation of danger, pain, and suffering is not what people of moral sensitivity tend to do. This inclination not to place people in jeopardy surely is a factor in declining birth rates during periods of adversity and in decisions to abort a pregnancy when the fetus is found to have a severe defect. Prospective parents routinely express a desire that their children be better off in life than they have been. This wish implies a willingness to do that which is necessary to maximize a child's opportunity. However, bringing hopes and dreams to reality may not always be easy or even possible.

It is estimated that sixteen out of every hundred ova exposed to spermatozoa fail to become fertilized. Of the eighty-four ova that are fertilized, representing potential births, only one-half (forty-two) are expected to survive in the womb beyond two weeks. The risk of embryonic death continues throughout pregnancy until at forty weeks only thirty-one of the original hundred possible births occur. The rate of pregnancy loss is substantial. Death of the embryo or fetus may result from intrinsic abnormalities that are fatal. Loss can also result from lethal environmental effects mediated via the female genital tract (due to the aging process, disease of the genital tract, or the transmission of exogenous teratogenic agents).[11] The death of infants adds to this trail of mortality (11.2/1,000 live births in 1982).[12] All things considered, becoming pregnant, bringing pregnancy to term, and the survival of the newborn for one year is a process filled with loss.

As indicated by rates of infant mortality, giving birth does not necessarily assure that the hopes and dreams associated with pregnancy will inevitably progress to realization. Approximately 7 percent of live-born infants have some form of birth defect.[13] (A compendium issued by the March of Dimes in 1979 lists 1,005 birth defects.) Some are reasonably insignificant, others are debilitating, and some are lethal.[14] (It is estimated that 60,000 deaths occur each year because of birth defects.[15]) Seven percent of births involve low birth weight infants,[16] a major cause of infant mortality and morbidity; around 4 percent of newborns have a readily detectable congenital anomaly.[17] Some will die in infancy, others will survive only to die prematurely. Perhaps as many as 30,000 babies are born each year so severely malformed that they will lead greatly circumscribed lives if they survive. And with survival comes the prospect that their medical care will extend far beyond the newborn period. The March of Dimes estimates that 1.2 million infants, children, and adults are hospitalized annually for the treatment of or for complications of birth defects.[18]

When a normal, healthy baby is born parental reactions tend to begin with relief. The lurking, unspoken worry that something could and might go wrong during pregnancy and birth is over. The hopes and dreams that accompanied pregnancy seem a bit more realistic. Announcements are made. Family and friends, ever mindful of the potential dangers in childbirth, inquire nervously if mother and child are well. When assured that they are the relief of the parents becomes theirs as well. The process of change and adjustment that began with the decision to conceive continues after birth.[19] Partners begin to adjust to their new roles as parents. They assume responsibility to provide the care and necessities their child needs for growth and development. New goals are fashioned and old goals are revised as necessary to accommodate their collective futures as mom, dad, and child.

The birth of an infant that requires medical care for a serious or prospective chronic problem tends to prompt a different sequence of responses. Two calamities must be faced. First, parents grieve the loss of the perfect imagined baby that was not born. Second, they must cope with the birth of the feared, threatening, anger-provoking defective infant that was born.[20] My observations are consistent with published reports regarding parental reactions to the birth of a diseased or defective newborn. The response may be generalized in the following way: When a new mother and father hears that "there are some problems with their baby" they tend to be shocked. Their reaction is shaped to a significant extent by the type and degree of defect, their past experiences, religious beliefs, values, and personalities. How a particular family adjusts is related to the customary ways with which it deals with stress.[21] Questions are asked: Can it be fixed? Is it visible? Does it affect the brain? The senses? Will he or she be paralyzed? Does it affect the genitalia? What effect will it have on future development? Disbelief is not uncommon. If the defect is internal, it is not unusual for parents to remark, when they first see the baby, "she is so pretty, I can't believe anything is wrong." Visible defects may contribute to parental shock and dispel disbelief. Parents are told of their child's problems and what to expect when they visit the baby in the nursery or intensive care unit. Nevertheless, they often imagine the appearance of their newborn to be worse than it actually is. The news that something is wrong may be more destabilizing than sight of the child. Shock and disbelief are only the first stages of a possibly long process of adjustment to an unexpected and, perhaps, unwanted child. Parental responses may be influenced by the appearance of the baby initially and by the baby's responses continually. A different future than the one anticipated has been set in motion.

Sadness, anger, anxiety, and fear may not be far behind shock and disbelief. The order of responses varies, and they do not necessarily progress to acceptance. They change during the course of hospitalization and, if the child survives, after discharge. Parents begin to reconcile the child of their fantasies with the one that was delivered. Explanations are sought. Why did this happen? How did this happen? Who is responsible? The mother may feel that she is to blame for the baby's condition. She may feel inadequate, concerned that she has failed her husband as well as their baby. The stress of the first days may be increased by a separation of the family. The mother may be in a maternity or general hospital, the baby in a specialized nursery in a different hospital (perhaps in a different city), and the father shuttles between two hospitals, work, and home. Mother and father may be protective of each other. They try to be strong, to mask their anxiety and fear, to be cautiously optimistic.

First visits may be poignant to observe, particularly if the baby is in an intensive care unit and the prognosis is not hopeful. Usually few words are spoken. An uneasy quiet envelops the immediate vicinity of the crib. Mom and dad usually are gowned. Arm-in-arm they are directed to their baby by one of the ICU personnel. The baby's nurse is introduced. The nurse is trained to be aware of parental concerns, to be supportive, and to encourage, when possible, their involvement in the baby's care. The infant may be motionless, paralyzed with drugs when placed on a respirator. The only movement is that of the rhythmic rise and fall of the baby's chest in response to a machine that supports its life. Tubes may be going into the body, sensors to monitor vital functions may be stuck on, and pads may cover his or her eyes. If very premature or deformed, the baby's appearance may not be pleasant. Parents tend to sit, cry, and stroke the baby, if possible. The parents who are optimistic about the prognosis tend to touch and talk to the baby. The body language of parents who are afraid and have little hope is revealing. They tend to stand or sit next to the crib with their heads slightly lowered.

Nurses report that parents seem fearful to ask questions that may bring an answer they don't want to hear. Indigent parents may be more timid in their questioning and will only question the nurse. Visiting may be less frequent because of a lack of transportation or bus fare. Regardless of these behaviors, the emotional reactions of indigent parents seem not to be remarkably different from parents in other social and economic classes. If they are able to hold the baby, tensions seem to ease. Comments tend to be "we'll do what we must for this baby" rather than "we can't deal with this baby." This description is representative of parental reactions during the first visit. By no means does it approach an adequate description of the highly individualized and varied first meeting of parents and sick newborn.

When survival is in doubt, naming may be delayed. Becoming someone other than Baby Boy Jones or Baby Girl Smith is significant. Naming personalizes; it expresses an attachment or bond between the one named and those who do the naming. Robert and Peggy Stinson have published excerpts from the journals they kept during the dying of their newborn son. Theirs is a revealing record of what can happen when a baby is born with something wrong. Andrew was delivered at twenty-four weeks weighing 28 ounces (800 grams). Peggy Stinson's notes concerning the naming of their son are thought provoking: "It's hard for other people to understand that Andrew is beginning to seem like a real baby to us. I feel more drawn to him now that I can think of him as having a name. Names that appeal to you in sound or look or association carry with them pleasant images and expectations. 'Marginally viable infant' was a negative, scary label, calling up visions of machinery and sterile rooms and someone not quite human. Andrew is a little blond boy with mischievous blue eyes crawling or running around the living room."[22] The son of her fantasy was not her son in the crib.

Parents often feel helpless in situations of critical illness or major defect. They may feel powerless to affect the life of the child. The child's needs are being met by others; nurses and doctors feed, change, hold, and protect the baby. Mom and dad may be able to only visit, stand by, and express their concern. They may be excluded from participating in decisions regarding every aspect of their baby's life. Again, the words of the Stinson's are telling: " . . . Carvalho [a neonatologist] had taken over the baby. He would treat the baby according to his ideas about what was right even though he could see that his moral or religious views differed drastically from ours. He could overrule us, could—and did—dismiss what we believe automatically, unemotionally, as if we were beneath notice. Because he has the power." The tenuous bond established with naming can be threatened by separation from the infant and discord with the medical team. Near the end of Andrew's life, Mrs. Stinson wrote: "I keep trying to puzzle out to what extent the Andrew in the IICU [infant intensive care unit] is *our responsibility*, is even our Andrew. His problems, his diseases and damage, are not continual but iatrogenic—caused by the inability of his doctors with their present knowledge and equipment (using treatment we did not specifically authorize) to safeguard his brain and other vital systems while they try to make him live and grow. Whatever abilities or disabilities he will have, what personality, even what physical stature will not be the traits of the original Andrew—what he started out with, in a sense, at conception, what he inherited from us—but the traits produced in the IICU. Andrew will be, in important ways, a person grown by scientists in a lab—if he's not 'turning out well' they're at least learning how to produce the next person a little better."[23] Perhaps no other scene is so desperate as one in which a mother, sensing a threat to her child, is impotent to shield the child from injury, or to comfort once the injury is sustained.

Efforts to "parent" may be expressed by visits to the baby and inquiries about his or her progress. Some mothers call the nursery each time they awake at night. One mother I know kept a narrative of her baby's course in a stenographer's notebook. Entries began, "They told my mother that. . . . " When asked about this she replied that it was painful to her but the baby would want to see it when she was older. The mother disclaimed wanting to read it herself. The main reason she kept the journal, according to her, was that it was the only method of control she had over the situation.

Laboratory values or respirator settings may become a preoccupation. Any and every sign for hope may be seized upon while the overall and long-term assessment may be carefully avoided. The placement of stuffed animals, tapes of parents speaking lovingly, Bibles, tape players with recordings of Bible verses, or other religious symbols in an infant's crib are tangible evidence of parental bonding with and hope for a newborn with a questionable future. If brought from home they represent a link to home. They express the parent's hope that the child will become normal. The significance of these symbols ought not be underestimated. Parents have searched the cribs of other infants, even notified the hospital administrator, when a toy, Bible, or some other symbol has been misplaced. I do not understand the full meaning of these symbols for parents, but I do appreciate them as genuine indications of attachment. In some instances, this may be one thing that parents can do while physicians and nurses do almost everything else for the infant.

The time may come when the parents' ambivalence about the destiny of their child is expressed. They may want the baby to live but not if pain and suffering is his or her fate. Wanting a baby to live and at the same time being prepared to accept a baby's death is a legitimate and common feeling for parents when the prognosis for a seriously ill baby is one of severe mental and physical handicap if he or she survives. To gloss over the impact of such a child on a family is naive. To wish a life of pain and suffering incommensurate with any joy or pleasure such a life may bring to the one who lives it is, at best, morally suspect.

The uncertainties that surround the birth of a defective or seriously ill newborn are not limited to the immediate family. Announcements of the birth may be deferred until a clearer assessment of the child's condition and future is known. The established customs of visitation and gifts seem awkward in these circumstances. Friends and family who otherwise would have been attentive may be silent and absent. Well-intentioned people may simply not want to risk saying something wrong that might compound the pain, anxiety, and embarrassment that parents may feel. Children with birth defects who endeavor to assume their place in society must cope with the social reaction to their defect. The response of others determines in many ways the effect of a congenital impairment on an individual. Many studies show that "normal" people tend to stigmatize and reject those who are "different." One result of this sort of social reaction may be isolation for the impaired individual and his or her family. The interaction that occurs is often on a superficial level. People seem to fear that they, too, will be stigmatized if they associate too closely with the family of the stigmatized individual.[24]

The burden of care between the time a child goes home and the age at which it begins school tends to be treated as a personal tragedy to be borne by the family, not a social burden to be borne collectively. The mothers of children born with deformities caused by the drug Thalidomide may be representative of mothers with comparably impaired infants. A Canadian study of these mothers reports that there was constant change and "what seemed lacking was any sense of teleology, or even continuity, in this change." Independence for the child and parent alike, however minimal, simply was beyond their grasp. Life had to be lived from one day to the next. In order to be able to perform maternal tasks, each woman had to recognize psychologically the similarities between her child and normal people as well as the differences. "It was because they [mothers] could see these children in their own image," the researchers reported, "that the multiple differences manifested could be assimilated and tolerated."[25]

The isolation from friends and estrangement from the child that may have begun while the child was in the hospital may continue after hospitalization. The hospital and medical bills arrive. Parents realize that survival carries a financial cost. Though a high percentage of these costs may be paid by insurance companies, families frequently must share in these payments. These expenses can literally bankrupt a family. Other stresses may come from the demands of the severely impaired or chronically ill infant on the family schedule. Feeding, crying, diapering, and nursing care may result in parents being perpetually fatigued. Each illness awakens or renews earlier feelings of guilt or fear and further worsens the family's financial situation. The slow and uneven development of the child can increase parental worries about the eventual capacities of the child.[26] Parents may develop a "chronic sorrow" that "may lie dormant and unnoticed for long periods of time only to surge forth unexpectedly. It may be simply looking out one's window to see a little girl skipping home from school on a crisp fall day, blithely kicking piles of red and yellow leaves which brings the almost forgotten tears to a parent's eyes months or years after all the tears were thought to have been shed."[27] Grief can turn into anger when parents recognize that they may never be free of this level of intense care. The anger may be directed against the child in the form of neglect, abuse, accidents, or failure to thrive.[28] Coping with the child's problems can lead to a major reorganization of family life. A point of equilibrium may be reached[29] in which parents may come to accept their situation. Their confidence in their ability to care for this child may increase. Some measure of peace, even pleasure, may be derived from this experience. But this point is not achieved without considerable cost to all concerned, if at all. Everything considered, it is understandable that some parents report feeling "trapped" when their baby survives with a severe physical or mental defect that precludes any possibility of the child becoming independent and their being liberated from a seemingless endless service to him or her.

This partial, general description of parental reactions to the birth of a baby with some kind of defect clearly does not capture all the ways in which parents respond to the adversity of a defective or low birth weight baby. I have attempted to portray how parents feel and behave when forced to come to terms with a possibility that was feared and has become a reality. The spectrum of reactions are too diverse and complex to be completely portrayed by the picture drawn here. The several actual case reports that follow show how individual parents have responded to reproductive adversity and the apparent or expressed bases upon which treatment decisions were made. These case reports are presented for illustrative purposes only. They are not meant as examples of good or bad moral decision making. The first case is perhaps the one most cited in published discussions of decision making in newborn medicine.[30]

A baby was born with Down syndrome complicated by a duodenal atresia (intestinal blockage). Without surgical repair of the blockage, a routine procedure with minimal risk, the baby could not be fed and would die. The mother was a thirty-four-year-old hospital nurse, the father a thirty-five-year-old lawyer. They had two other children. The parents refused the surgical repair of the blockage indicating that it would be unfair to the other children to raise them with a Down syndrome sibling. The uncertain extent of mental retardation associated with Down syndrome children was explained to the parents by the physician. These children were described as trainable (in most cases), employable in simple jobs, and capable of a long life, provided there were no significant complications. Nevertheless, the parents refused to consent to surgery and the physicians agreed with the parents' decision. The fact that the child would be mentally retarded, at an unknown and unpredictable level, was deemed by parents and physicians alike as a sufficient reason to utilize a different standard for treatment decisions. Life, according to the physicians, tends to be valued on the basis of intelligence. With this future unknown, the parents' instructions were followed. The child was placed in a side room, not fed, and died several days later. The basis upon which life-sustaining treatment was refused in this case report is most obviously the baby's anticipated neurological and/or mental incapacity. But the prospect of mental impairment may not be the only reason that life-prolonging treatment may be refused.

Another criterion was used by a Mexican migrant worker. The man's wife gave birth to a premature baby with a severe, and probably fatal, respiratory disorder. In addition, the baby had micro-penis, which is usually treated by the surgical removal of the nonfunctional genitals. The child is then raised as a female. The father of this baby felt very threatened by the sexual inadequacy of his son. Rather than cope with a perceived failure of his masculinity, the father, with the consent of the mother, refused treatment of the infant's respiratory disease. Treatment, nevertheless, was undertaken but the baby died anyway. As this case report makes evident, the defect need not be visible to others or affect the brain in order to provoke a judgment that death of the newborn is a desirable end.

Another form of parental response is found in the case of a baby boy born to a seventeen-year-old, unmarried woman. This was her first pregnancy. She decided prior to delivery to place the child for adoption. The delivery was normal and the child was placed with adoptive parents through an agency. The adoptive parents were named conservators by a judge prior to the completion of the adoption. On day ten of life, the adoptive parents noticed lesions on the child's shoulder. The next day the infant was taken to a local emergency room where a diagnosis of a possible staph infection or chicken pox was made. The infant was sent home and apparently did well for several days. On day seventeen of life, the adoptive parents decided that the infant seemed too sleepy and lethargic for everything to be fine. On day eighteen, in the early evening, the baby developed difficulty breathing. He was taken to another hospital's emergency room where he was treated, admitted, placed on antibiotics and monitored. Within five hours the baby was transferred to a neonatal intensive care unit in, now, a third hospital. A diagnosis of herpes encephalitis of unknown source was made. The baby developed additional neurological, cardiac, and respiratory problems.

The chance for survival of the infant, if given proper treatment, was estimated at 50 percent. If he survived, the physicians estimated that he would be severely retarded having a possible I.Q. of 50 or less. Institutionalization was probable because of his neurological, pulmonary, and other likely chronic problems. The burden of care was considered too great for the parents to provide without special equipment and outside of a specialized setting. The adoptive parents had one other child by adoption. They expressed deep concern about the condition and future of this child. Even though not yet legally his adoptive parents, they considered the newborn to be their responsibility. They consulted their pastor about the situation. They visited the baby regularly, talked, smiled, and handled him. Even though their desires for a healthy infant were frustrated, they expressed a moral obligation to maintain their responsibility for this child. The ICU personnel believed that the adoptive parents had become sufficiently attached to the infant to be unable to return the child to the court's custody.

The medical and nursing staffs had intense feelings about this infant and adoptive parents. They perceived the parents as kind, generous, and self-sacrificing people being unfairly burdened by this infant. As a result, the medical and nursing personnel tended to be less aggressive with their treatment, hoping that the child would die and relieve the adoptive parents of this injustice. After all, the father was a factory worker on a limited income. The long-term care of this infant would require a considerable investment of money and time. Some of the medical personnel felt that the other adoptive child and these parents should be protected from the burden this child represented.

We must resist an extended discussion of the propriety of the medical and nursing preferences in this case. For example, Was the felt need to protect the adoptive parents warranted? Should treatment decisions for children who remain with their biological parents be different from decisions made for infants placed for adoption? The adoptive parents in this case clearly were prepared to accept the burden of care as part of their moral obligations to this child, independent of the source or nature of his illness. The adoption had not been completed. The child could have been returned to the court's jurisdiction. Doing so would have relieved this couple of all financial and legal obligations to or in behalf of this child. But despite the feeling of others that they ought not to have to bear this burden, the couple persisted in their desire to proceed with the adoption. Even though they had not received what they had expected, and a direct bond between them and this infant was not established during the course of pregnancy, the man and woman maintained their readiness to continue in the parental role for this child regardless of the emotional and financial costs.

The parents' desire to keep this baby when they could have chosen otherwise, and when their decision cast them in a perpetual maintenance role for this child, might be considered above and beyond all reasonable requirements. On the other hand, the response of the parents of the child with Down syndrome and intestinal blockage has been criticized by many commentators as selfish. The great majority of responses, in my experience, involve parental efforts to consider all factors and make a judgment that appears to serve the most good. The following case is an example of this sort of response.

An infant was born to a woman in her late twenties. She and her husband have a two-year-old child. The parents describe themselves as faithful Roman Catholics. The current pregnancy resulted in the delivery of an infant with multiple anomalies. The baby had an exposed urinary bladder, mild fluid buildup in the head, ambiguous genitalia, a spine disconnected from the pelvis, no anus, agenesis of the colon, and a meningocele (sac containing membranes and fluid) at the base of the spine. Urine and stools were excreted onto the exposed urinary bladder. This made feeding difficult since waste excreted onto the exposed bladder increased the risk of infection. The baby had a normal small bowel, kidneys, heart, and lungs. Multiple specialists were consulted about possible treatments. The baby was found to be chromosomally male (XY), but because of the nonfunctional status of his genitalia, it was recommended that the infant be considered female, named appropriately, and raised accordingly, if the infant survived. Abdominal surgical options included a diverting colostomy to prevent the bowel from emptying onto the exposed bladder, followed by surgical efforts to enclose the bladder within the body. The meningocele was unsightly; however, any surgery on the sac was considered more cosmetic than therapeutic. There was no immediate need to provide a shunt or drain for the mild fluid buildup in the head since it was believed to be draining through the spinal column into the meningocele. In addition, surgery on the sac was not expected to restore function to the infant's legs, which had atrophied in the womb.

The initial request by the parents was that everything should be done. They said that they had wanted this pregnancy and baby very much. As additional diagnostic data were obtained and a more complete clinical picture became available, the prognosis for the infant began to qualify their initial treatment requests. The possible surgeries to collect urine and stools in ostomy bags would have made management of the child easier but would not have affected the child's mental and relational capacities. Mild to severe mental retardation was projected. Efforts to redirect the draining of the hydrocephalus would require surgery initially every three months or so. Again, these procedures were not believed to affect the ultimate outcome but would have helped to decrease the expansion of the meningocele. If the baby survived, which was by no means certain, the medical opinion was that the patient would be wheelchair-bound. Eventually, the child would develop severe scoliosis (curvature of the spine), which meant that ultimately the patient would be bound to a bed.

The parents' religious beliefs were a major factor in how they viewed this infant and their responsibilities for it. The paternal grandmother held an advanced degree in theology from a Roman Catholic university. After extensive consultation with the physicians and the grandmother, the parents decided that all of the surgical options were extraordinary, and therefore not required by canons of moral theology or indicated by the total clinical description of the infant. They decided that nursing care was ordinary care and, therefore, all that was required. The antibiotics that were being given were discontinued. Efforts to feed orally were attempted but unsuccessful and so intravenous nutrition was continued. Within a few days the infant died of a chemical imbalance even though efforts were made to treat it. After the infant died the family expressed satisfaction with the care the baby and they received. They stated that their decisions regarding treatment were made by considering the prognosis of the infant alone. The prospective impact of this child on the family was not given primary importance during the course of their deliberations. They tended to focus on the infant, the sort of life the baby would have if he survived, and the cost to the child in terms of pain, suffering, and handicap necessary to prolong survival. In essence, they concluded that the path of surgical treatment would not offer a reasonable prospect for benefit to the child and would involve excessive pain, suffering, and expense.[31] Reaching this decision involved considerable anguish on the part of the parents. Their desires, coupled with their religious convictions, disposed them to a different judgment. But when all of the evidence was gathered, they sought to protect the child in the way they considered best, sacrificing their hopes and dreams for this baby. Their assessment was that the costs to the infant of its prolonged survival defeated their parental duties to seek its continued life by extraordinary means.

Another case in which religious commitments did not play a role involved a baby born with nonfunctional kidneys. The baby was also asphyxiated (receiving no oxygen) at birth, which was anticipated to lead to a mild mental retardation. The baby could survive but would require regular dialysis treatments until a kidney transplant could be obtained. The parents were reflective people. They had a second child, described as a toddler, at home. Like the parents in the preceding case, this couple focused on the prognosis for the child as their primary consideration. But unlike the preceding case, these parents also expressed concern about the impact the care of this infant would have on the family, especially the development and opportunity of the child at home. They chose not to seek long-term renal dialysis for this baby. It could not cure the infant and the procedure itself carried risks that could lead to a quick death. Neither would dialysis reverse the anticipated mental retardation. The parents also understood the care requirements necessary to maintain the newborn's life. In the end, they determined that they could not personally meet the long-term requirements. Their joint income was small. They lived modestly and were concerned with providing the best opportunity for their children that they could. In short, this baby endangered all that they had worked toward as husband and wife, and as a family. They also judged that the infant's quality of life, understood in terms of what the infant could experience and what would be necessary to maintain life, did not warrant pursuing renal dialysis. The mother imagined herself in the infant's situation. She commented, "If I were him, I wouldn't want to go through all of this. I wouldn't want it done to me." The parents subsequently were able to take the baby home to die.

Why parents respond to crises in the way they do depends on multiple variables particular to the individuals involved. The range of responses reflect unique personal and family histories. The varied responses, insofar as they are influenced by moral values, beliefs, and norms, also provide evidence of the moral pluralism in which we live. This observation is illustrated by the expressed preferences, the goods pursued, the harms avoided, the weighing of benefits and burdens, the ranking of interests, the assessment of duties and obligations implicit in these abbreviated case reports. Some parents value an infant's life over all other considerations. Other parents attempt to balance the anticipated good of life to a newborn against the probable losses or harms to the family that are related to the costs of sustaining the infant. Some parents separate their duties toward an imperiled neonate from their duties toward other children. Other parents consider their duties toward one child to be conditioned by their duties toward other children in the home. Some parents are disposed to alter plans and dreams to accommodate the special needs of a chronically ill or defective infant. Other parents are disposed only to receive into their home an infant whose probable future is compatible with the one they imagined for their family. Parents decide for or against life-prolonging interventions for reasons as varied as the people themselves. The facts and circumstances of any given case when refracted through the lens of different moralities can lead to multiple licit understandings of what is morally required or allowed. This suggests that efforts to legislate or regulate the medical care of newborns in a way that gives proper regard to these variables will be difficult, if not impossible.

The propositions that (1) parents are primarily responsible for making decisions regarding the medical care of an imperiled newborn, and that (2) decisions for or against life-prolonging treatment can properly be based in part on the probability that the infant can attain independence, are strengthened by the perspective of the contemporary family and parenting as shown in the case histories. Special care for a perpetually dependent child may diminish the quality of family life insofar as quality is determined by foregone opportunities and benefits. Parents are uniquely situated to consider the newborn's condition and probable future in relation to their circumstances and moral commitments. Similarly, they are positioned to assess the probable effect the infant will have on the quality of family life.

Contemporary patterns of family formation and family size suggest, among other things, an enhanced concern for the quality of life. Respect for the notion of the quality of family life seems implicit in public approval of contraception and abortion. This is true particularly if the quality of family life is related to the number of pregnancies and births. Prenatal diagnosis and abortion allows couples to limit the potentially destructive impact that an abnormal or unhealthy baby could have on their family. Parental authority to act defensively with regard to the potential burden of a chronically dependent child ought not to be limited to the prenatal period because concern for the quality of family life is not restricted to this period. Neither should the ability of parents to make treatment decisions for an imperiled newborn on quality-of-family-life criteria be restricted to the prenatal period. Parental authority in this regard properly ought to extend at least through the neonatal period (twenty-eight days) for infants with a high probability to significantly, and perhaps unjustly, limit the opportunities and benefits of other family members. This argument for extended parental control ought not to be understood to endorse a disregard for the value of life to the infant. The infant's perceived quality of life is an important factor to consider. But it is only one among other perhaps equally weighty, depending on one's point of view, factors. The integrity of the family is a value and is valued in contemporary society. Similarly, improving the quality of life for the family unit and its individual members tends to be a goal for parents. Accordingly, the authority and power of parents to govern their family, to define the meaning of quality for themselves, and to act to promote those ends in morally permissible ways ought not to be compromised unnecessarily by other individuals or the state.

The effect on parents and family of a baby born prematurely, malformed, or defective varies widely. The observations and case reports provided above indicate a range of attitudes, adjustments, and responses to the birth of an infant with severe problems. Parents are uniquely situated to know the goals and values of the family. As such, they are better able than anyone else to assess the impact an impaired infant will have on the family and, as importantly, their ability to provide the special care an impaired infant requires. Parents seem, according to my observations, to evidence genuine and balanced concern for the fate of their healthy or unhealthy newborn. In the vast majority of instances, parents who must deal with the misfortune of an impaired infant respond conscientiously, seeking to do the best as they understand it for the infant and others immediately involved (e.g., themselves and their other children). As I stated in Chapter 1, parents are required to make only reasonable decisions. At times parents may make decisions on grounds or for reasons that appear suspect to people who embrace different moral values, pursue different valid goals, and favor other legitimate means to attain them. Such is the nature of a moral pluralism. Respect for reasonable parental judgments honors the value of the integrity of the family and serves the best interests of children as a class. In essence, parents have a fiduciary role. They have the primary responsibility to weigh the probable risks and rewards of decisions affecting the welfare and well-being of their children. These assessments are frequently influenced by a concern for the family as a viable entity. Parents are in a position of authority and power, responsible for their child during his or her dependency, and obliged to facilitate the child's independence where independence is possible. Functioning as a trustee, parents are expected to discern a child's interest both as an individual and in the contexts of the family and society of which he or she is a part.

Parents as Quasi-Trustees

The image of parents as the trustees of a child's interests is not unprecedented. We found in Chapter 2, in the discussion of the status of children, that John Locke, Martin Luther, and the tradition of law utilized some form of the notion of trust to express their respective understandings of the parent-child relation. John Locke and Martin Luther held that parental authority is exercised in trust under God for the good or benefit of a child. The law presumes that parents are worthy of the trust to properly perform the duties assigned to them. This presumption is basic to its support of parental authority and respect for the integrity of the family. Finally, Luther, Locke, and the law agree that the duty and authority of parents are related both to the ends sought in parenting and to the ends sanctioned by the relevant superior authority (the moral community or God). These precedents can be construed as three principles of the trust relation of parent and child that guide and limit parental discretion: the good or benefit of a child is a primary concern; the trustee (parent) is to act in a responsible manner to promote legitimate ends; and legitimate ends are internal to the task of child-rearing (e.g., independence) and subject to external approval (i.e., standard of reasonableness).

When these principles are placed in the context of a morally pluralistic society, an image or model of parenting that is analogous to trust relationships can be constructed. A trusteelike image or model of parenting illuminates the nature of the parent-child relation and suggests the boundaries of parental discretion. In speaking of parents as *"quasi*-trustees" or of having *"quasi*-fiduciary"* authority, I am signaling the similarities and dissimilarities of the roles of parent and trustee. I intend to evoke an image or model that illuminates parental authority and duty. I do not intend, nor do I believe that it is possible except in the most general way, to stipulate how parents ought to fulfill their role duties toward an imperiled newborn. These decisions are properly individualized, conditioned by the medical facts, family circumstances, and moral commitments of parents. Accordingly, the standard of reasonableness has been advocated to establish the limits of parental discretion in these cases.

Certain features of the fiduciary role of parents that I endorse can be drawn from the law. The parental role vis-à-vis children is analogous to the role of trustees vis-à-vis a beneficiary. A trustee holds something for another's benefit. Thus a bank may hold a depositor's money for his or her benefit, e.g., safety or appreciation through prudent investment. In like manner, a parent holds discretionary authority for the benefit of a child or, according to some commmentators, the state or God. In a sense, parents can be said to have a triple agency: They are to make judgments that advance the interests of a child, the family, and the society of which they are members. Not an easy assignment.

In a trust relation there is a separation of interests. The property of the trust is not the property of the trustee even though the trustee may be empowered to make decisions regarding its use or disposition. The trustee is not usually allowed to use the property in a trust for his or her own benefit. Rather, the trustee's sole, legitimate interest in the relation is the performance of the

duties identified in the document creating the trust. The trust in-
denture defines the authority considered necessary for the trustee
to achieve the purposes for which the trust was created. Without
this sort of separation of interests, a trust would not be necessary.

In the same way, a child is not the property of parents. Their
identities are separable. Their interests may be separable. I have
argued that the interests of a child are properly related to and
understood in the context of his or her family. This relation, however, does not necessarily establish or confer upon parents the
right to disregard or deny the legitimate interests of a child, however they are ascertained. It would be difficult, perhaps impossible, for anyone other than those individuals, primarily parents,
with intimate and informed knowledge of a child to begin to
stipulate a child's interests except in a general manner. The particular circumstances of child, family, and society are too variable
to allow for any specification of interests other than the formal
interests of independence and enrichment. These interests may
be served by the provision, for example, of education, preventive
and curative medical care, nutrition, safety, and employment.
Parents in a trusteelike role are responsible to use their experience
and knowledge to identify a child's interests. They are responsible to use their authority and power to facilitate a child's interests understood formally as liberation or independence and
enrichment. In cases where parents intentionally or unintentionally disregard, or misperceive, the child's interests and make unreasonable decisions or act in unreasonable ways, they properly
may be restrained from imposing unwarranted harms on a child.
Parents who make good faith but wrong judgments deserve cor-
rection and instruction. They do not forfeit their customary parental authority because of honest mistakes. Parents who are
intentionally malevolent toward a child may have their authority
removed by the moral community and state because they have
forfeited the trust that was placed in them. Stated differently, they
have acted unreasonably.

A legal trust usually is limited in duration and can be set aside
by the terms of the trust, by agreement, or by a court order. Similarly, by law and custom parental responsibility and authority are
usually limited to the period of a child's dependency, i.e., minority in nearly all instances. During this period, performance by
the trustee can be enforced by legal and/or social sanctions. Marriage or parenting may emancipate a child from parental author-

ity, depending on the legal jurisdiction and local custom. Or a judge may terminate parental custody, control, and responsibility in favor of a surrogate when cause is shown. But as long as a trustee acts in good faith and within the limits established by the law, the trustee's discretion is unhindered. Such tends to be the case with parental discretion. As long as parents act honestly and with primary and genuine concern for the welfare and well-being of a child, exercises of express and implied powers tend not to be challenged.

Parents are entrusted with power and authority over a specific period of their child's life, the period of minority or dependence. Like trustees in law, parents are bound to exercise due care, diligence, and skill in the performance of their duties and in the exercise of their authority. The legal standard of performance for a trustee is what an ordinarily prudent person would do in the conduct of his private affairs in a similar circumstance and with a similar object in view. "Whether or not a trustee meets the standard or measure of care required of him depends on circumstances as they exist at the time that he acts, and not upon subsequent developments. Wisdom developed after an event, and having it and its consequences as its source, is a standard by which no man should be judged."[32] Thus, a result unfavorable to the interest of the beneficiary does not necessarily indicate that the trustee was guilty of gross negligence or mismanagement. Similarly, the standard for judgment of parental actions or decisions regarding a child must take into consideration the circumstances at the time the action or decision occurred. Actions or decisions concerning the medical care of a child should be evaluated on the basis of what is reasonably known and anticipated at the time. Hindsight is the only perfect vision. Unanticipated weal or woe does not legitimate or condemn necessarily a good faith and reasonable action or decision. In short, parents ought to consider all available relevant information and act or decide on a reasoned assessment of that information. To the extent that this is done, they have performed their duty and exercised their responsibility adequately.

As mentioned, a trust relation can be terminated by the terms of the trust document, by agreement, or by a court order. A trust also may be terminated if performance of the trust is impossible. Assume that a trustee is obligated to operate an oil lease for the benefit of a religious institute. If the oil well becomes totally de-

pleted the trustee can no longer execute the terms of the trust.
The trust relation between trustee and beneficiary could be terminated. Assume that the religious institute becomes a Sunday
School or a seminary. This change in the condition of the beneficiary is not necessarily a sufficient cause to terminate the trust.
So long as it remains the same legal entity and fulfills the same
basic function the trust endures. In the case of parents and a seriously ill newborn, the parents' obligations to maintain and nurture toward independence may be impossible to fulfill—the child
may have a terminal condition; death may be imminent. But the
parental obligations to manage the child do not cease. They take
a different form and serve a different immediate goal. The duty
to protect from pain and suffering may take priority over a duty
to prolong life. When the child dies, the existential relation ends.
The trust ends.

Two types of changes in a child's condition, other than death,
can terminate the fiduciarylike responsibility of a parent: majority
and emancipation by law (e.g., marriage, giving birth) or custom
(e.g., self-support). A change in an infant's medical condition
short of death does not terminate the trust or parent-child relation
and correlate duties. That a healthy child becomes ill in and of
itself does not relieve parents of their duties toward a child. To
the contrary, duties to care are even greater in response to the
threat of illness. But when a child's medical condition changes
from curable to inescapably terminal the duties to care may be
expressed differently. The prospect of the imminent death of a
child necessarily redefines the ends parental duties are to serve.
Independence is forever denied to the child. The achievable goals
for this fading life become limited. In addition, the alternative
ways by which these limited objectives can be sought become
fewer. Nevertheless, the relation between parent and child endures. The parents remain primarily responsible for the child,
empowered to make decisions and to take actions for the benefit
of the child, however reasonably interpreted in the circumstances.

A trustee may be displaced for violating his or her role as
guardian.[33] Reckless and imprudent management of the principal
of a trust may be grounds to remove a trustee. Analogously, cruel
treatment or malicious neglect of a child may warrant taking custody and control of a child from the parents. Overriding a parent's decision or action is not indicated in normal circumstances

unless there is a willful parental failure to provide the necessities of life, including *routine* medical care that will restore a child to his or her former state, or preserve him or her at a level compatible with independence. Otherwise parental judgments ought to stand.

Parents, like trustees in law, should be worthy of the trust that has been placed in them. Their presumed knowledge and experience imposes upon them special obligations to make judgments that intend a dependent child's well-being. Like professionals, or legal trustees, parents define and interpret reality. In life situations, options are included and excluded on the basis of an understanding of the situation and context. The relevant and potential goods and harms expected to follow a decision or action are evaluated. Throughout this process of sorting through rules and anticipating consequences, parents, in order not to unnecessarily risk harm, injury, or wrong for a child or their family, ought not to lose sight of a key objective; the welfare and well-being of a child understood minimally in terms of a capacity for independence. Insofar as parents intend and reasonably facilitate this end, to the degree that they are able, their trustworthiness is exhibited. Being trustworthy, then, is a basic moral requirement for parents or any other person who has authority to make decisions on behalf of and for the benefit of another.[34]

The right and freedom of prospective parents to control their reproduction by contraception and abortion should be extended to embrace a right and freedom, not to mention duty, to control their individual and family future through the responsible, considered exercise of their fiduciarylike authority to make reasonable decisions regarding the medical care of a defective newborn. Certainly parents can voluntarily abdicate or forfeit their responsibility, in which case others can assume the parental role. In other instances, parents rightly may have their liberty to act and decide removed when their conduct poses an unreasonable danger to a child. For example, when a parent refuses an established, nonexperimental medical treatment the absence of which would result in the death of a child who otherwise would be expected to become capable of independence.

This brief discussion of a model of parental duty and authority was not meant to detail what parents should decide or even how they should make decisions. It promotes a particular way of thinking about parenting and parental responsibilities. The welfare and well-being of children and the family, in the short and long term, are seen as corollary to the emphasis on independence in the last chapter.

I have argued herein that quality-of-life considerations have a significant influence on family decisions. A concern for quality applies to the couple, each child, and the family unit. The ordering of life, including the control of reproduction, is a means by which a desired quality of life can be pursued. The authority of parents to govern the potentially destructive impact of a reproductive defect ought not to be limited to the prenatal period. In making treatment decisions for diseased or defective newborns, it is proper for parents to consider more than the value of life to the newborn. They should balance the interests of the infant with the interests of other children and the family unit. The choice in these situations is not between two competing equals except in some abstract sense. The differences between a severely impaired neonate and healthy siblings, for example, are relevant. They were not created by the parents; rather, nature altered the equation. Thus it is not unfair to choose the interests of the healthy over the interests of the imperiled. The differences can be significant and a preference for the newborn might unjustly limit the opportunities and benefits of other family members. Further, a preference to safeguard the interests of family members does not always mean that the interests of the imperiled newborn are abridged. It may be in the newborn's interest that life-prolonging interventions are foregone. In some cases, the pain and suffering of continued existence may not be balanced by the pleasure of living.

Perceiving parents in a fiduciary role with respect to their children allows for a range of individual responses to reproductive misfortune. Unless parents are absent, choose unreasonably, or otherwise forfeit the trust placed in them to nurture children, their decisions for or against life-prolonging treatment for newborns with severe disease or defect deserve respect.

4

Neonatal Medicine: A Context of Intersecting Interests

T HE CAPABILITY OF PARENTS to exercise their responsibility for the medical care of a severely ill or defective newborn has been limited in the past because of the inadequacies of medicine. Before the twentieth century, infants born with lethal defects died when the condition ran its natural course. Some malformed infants who otherwise might have had some length of survival were killed intentionally or placed in situations in which an early death was a reasonable certainty. Medicine, for all practical purposes, was impotent to effectively intervene to rescue life or transform a sick baby into a healthy one. Parents necessarily received what the natural lottery of human reproduction delivered. Cure and/ or habilitation to a normal life were beyond the control of both the parents and medicine.

This situation began to change dramatically immediately prior to the present century. Some conditions of birth became more subject to medical manipulation. With medical assistance, parents have gradually, over the years, become able to exercise responsibility for compromised infants as medicine's power to prolong life and correct defects has increased. Advances in the medical care of newborns have been most remarkable during the past twenty-five years. Life, death, or handicap are no longer always subject to the vicissitudes of nature's will alone. As a result, parents and physicians are more accountable for the lives or deaths of newborns who heretofore would have died regardless of medical attempts to save them. An extension of parental and medical control into the first twenty-eight days of life, and even before that, into the womb, entails a commensurate extension of responsibility for decisions made during this period that influence or determine the physical destiny of newborns.

Given a capability to intervene when faced with a defective newborn, parents, physicians, and society are forced to make choices regarding whether and to what extent to intervene. Interests other than those of the infant warrant consideration. The interrelationships of life are such that any choice, for example to save with severe handicap or to accept death, will have an effect on the lives and futures of others. Whereas in the past these decisions essentially were private, today the reckoning of competing interests is more public as these babies have been removed from the confines of the home to be in the custodial care of physicians and hospitals. In order to place in perspective the context in which decisions regarding the medical care of severely defective newborns are made, this chapter surveys some modern medical developments that contributed to the creation of a pediatric subspecialty for newborns. The resultant context in which care is provided to critically ill or severely defective newborns is described as one in which potentially conflicting interests are expressed and negotiated. The role of the neonatologist, or more inclusively the full treatment team, and other potential decision makers in these difficult circumstances is examined.

Evolution of a Subspecialty

Medical interest in the care of the newborn has long roots. Soranus's text on gynecology from the early second century represents the practice of obstetrics and gynecology at its peak in the ancient world. In the section "On the Care of the Newborn," Soranus provides short, summary instructions concerning severing the umbilicial cord, swaddling and cleaning, bedding, feeding, weaning, teething, and potential "mishaps" during the newborn period. But prior to addressing these more or less routine issues, he first explains "How to Recognize the Newborn That Is Worth Rearing." His counsel deserves full expression.

> Now the midwife, having received the newborn, should first put
> it upon the earth, having examined beforehand whether the in-

fant is male or female, and should make an announcement by signs as is the custom of women. She should also consider whether it is worth rearing or not. And the infant which is suited by nature for rearing will be distinguished by the fact that its mother has spent the period of pregnancy in good health, for conditions which require medical care, especially those of the body, also harm the fetus and enfeeble the foundations of its life. Second, by the fact that it has been born at the due time, best at the end of nine months, and if it so happens, later; but also after only seven months. Furthermore by the fact that when put on the earth it immediately cries with proper vigor; for one that lives for some length of time without crying, or cries only weakly, is suspected of behaving so on account of some unfavorable condition. Also by the fact that it is perfect in all its parts, members and senses; that its ducts, namely of the ears, nose, pharynx, urethra, anus are free from obstruction; that the natural functions of every [member] are neither sluggish nor weak; that the joints bend and stretch; that it has due size and shape and is properly sensitive in every respect. This we may recognize from pressing the fingers against the surface of the body, for it is natural to suffer pain from everything that pricks or squeezes. And by conditions contrary to those mentioned, the infant not worth rearing is recognized.[1]

These ancient instructions contain several insights worth noting. First, Soranus recognized a link, the details of which were not fully understood apparently, between maternal health and the birth of a viable infant. Though not specified, certain conditions or events during pregnancy must have been related, accurately or not, to an abnormal development in utero. Second, the attention given to the length of gestation reflects an observation that a minimal gestation is necessary for a fetus to develop sufficiently in order to survive outside of the womb. Third, the tests for strength and function were not technological or sophisticated by contemporary standards, but they were believed adequate to forecast those infants able and worthy to survive and those not so well situated. The fatal judgment for those who failed to pass the tests may seem harsh or ill-considered from our perspective, but it represents the cultural opinion of the ancient world regarding newborns observed to be less than fully normal, acknowledging the therapeutic impotency of medicine. Maternal health, length of gestation, form, and function remain, even today, significant indicators of survivability and quality of life.

Needless to say, knowledge of prenatal development, new-born physiology, pathology, and therapeutics has advanced significantly beyond the insights of Soranus. Concentration on the newborn and attention to reducing the incidence of infant mortality during the modern era has yielded a wealth of understanding and curative power—and neonatology, a subspecialty in pediatrics devoted to the care of the newborn's first twenty-eight days of life. Modern interest in the care of the newborn is traceable to Pierre Budin, a French obstetrician. In 1892, he established the first consultation for nurselings (a counterpart to a well-baby clinic) at Charité Hospital in Paris. Budin focused on the basic problems of prematurity: temperature, feeding, and the diseases that accompany early birth. Budin utilized a warm-air incubator for premature infants (developed by E. S. Tarnier, another French obstetrician, in 1880) to keep these babies warm. With regard to feeding, he advocated breast or forced feeding in an amount of slightly more than 20 percent of the infant's body weight each day. In addition, he took several precautions to guard against infection. He separated healthy, sick, and suspect infants from one another, milk was heated prior to feedings, bottles of milk were kept cool in the summer, and wet nurses were required to wash before feedings. He published his treatment principles in *The Nurseling* (1907), the first four chapters of which were on infants with "congenital feebleness," usually due to premature labor. He was the first to classify infants as small or large for gestational age, observing that the large do poorly and the small seem never to rest.[2]

Both Budin and Tarnier had a student named Martin A. Couney. Couney is one of the more colorful figures in the history of newborn medicine. Budin asked Couney to exhibit a modified Tarnier incubator at the World Exposition in Berlin in 1896. Couney agreed and arranged to have live premature infants placed within them. A similar exhibit took place in London in 1897. It was described in the British medical journal, *Lancet:* "The main feature of this new incubator is the fact that it requires no constant and skilled care. It works automatically; both ventilation and heat are maintained without any fluctuations whatsoever, not only for hours, but even for days. The incubator need not be touched for these purposes, and the only attendance necessary is that needed for feeding and washing the infant. . . . Only air taken outside the building is supplied to the infant within the incubator. When we consider how often private houses, and even hospital wards, are inefficiently ventilated, it is not necessary to insist on the advantage of deriving the air-supply direct from the street or garden. . . . ''[3] The building that housed the London exhibit was divided into three sections. One section contained sleeping quarters for the wet nurse and supervisor. The opposite section was the nursery, housing the incubators and premature babies. The middle section was open to the public where the incubating babies could be observed. Couney brought the exhibit to the United States in 1903. It was shown annually at Coney Island as a sideshow attraction. A fee was charged and barkers were used to entice people to attend. The exhibit at Coney Island closed in 1943 after New York City opened its first premature infant station at Cornell's New York Hospital. Couney said, ''I made propaganda for the preemie. My work is done.''[4]

Chicago in 1914 was one of the cities across the United States where Couney took the incubator–premature infant exhibit. Soon afterward Julius Hess, an obstetrician, established a premature-infant center at Michael Reese Hospital. An innovator himself, Hess adopted and extended the treatment principles worked out by Budin. He devised a primitive transport system to move a baby from its place of delivery, usually in the home attended by midwife, to a special care nursery by modifying a physician's bag into a carrying case. He was later able to improve upon this system by persuading some taxicab owners to install an electrical outlet in their dashboards that would allow incubators to be used instead of a physician's case. Another of Hess's innovations was to bring high-risk mothers into the hospital to deliver their babies. Beds were set aside for these women, thus reducing the dangers to the infant associated with transport. Hess began a training program and other centers were established around the country by people who visited the facility at Reese Hospital.[5]

The story of the medical care of neonates in the twentieth century is an interesting account of medical curiosity and technological sophistication. From its former days of virtual impotence, newborn medicine has evolved to where it is able to offer the newborn almost all of the same services that are offered to older children and adults. Whereas dramatic, effective rescue was unusual during the first four weeks of life, now it is commonplace. Clement Smith, emeritus professor of pediatrics at Harvard Medical School, remembers the days before the specialization of newborn care when if a baby had difficulty breathing, was immature, of low birth weight, or had a structural or neurological abnormality, the immediate concern was survival. The quality of survival was an important concern but it was a secondary luxury. In those less powerful days, Smith writes, "if we could not produce immediately effective respiration and circulation, our cautious assistance was aimed essentially at keeping the infant from dying until he could make the physiological readjustment necessary to continue as a living infant instead of a physiologically displaced fetus. This he could usually do more effectively, and probably with less attendant risk than we could do for him."[6] In short, efforts were made to stabilize the baby so that it could declare itself a survivor or nonsurvivor. With increasingly effective care, this basic objective of special nurseries to provide better care for infants with acute illness has expanded to include another goal of pushing back viability, i.e., to save the lives of smaller and shorter gestation babies. Now that babies who earlier would have died are surviving, more problems to which they are prone are being observed, investigated, and treated. And the field of neonatology grows accordingly. There are now approximately 200 training programs in neonatology, approximately 600 hospitals with neonatal intensive care units, and approximately 7,500 neonatal intensive care beds.[7] These data depict a remarkable expansion of services that reflect not only medical but also public interest in the medical care of newborns.

Research in the first half of this century on the pathology, physiology, clinical observations, growth, and outcomes of premature infants set the stage for the transformation of quiet centers for newborns into intensive care units during the 1950s and 1960s. Pediatricians rather than obstetricians began to provide more care to newborns. Technological developments enabled high-risk newborns to receive better care. The drug culture of the 1960s contributed to a greater appreciation of the relation of maternal drug use to infant malformation and illness. Respirators were used more widely and new diseases were seen as infants began to survive (e.g., necrotizing enterocolitis, bronchopulmonary dysplasia, patent ductus arteriosus). Insurance and governmental coverage for the medical care of newborns expanded. The first calls for a neonatology subspecialty were heard. And three kinds of facilities were established to care for infants. In Level I nurseries, care is given to normal newborns, risks are assessed, and transitional care is provided (85 percent of pregnancies). In Level II nurseries, in addition to offering the services of Level I units, care is provided for the moderately ill or recovering neonate (12 percent of pregnancies). Finally, in addition to the care available in Level I and II nurseries, any complication of pregnancy or neonatal illness can be treated in Level III units (intensive care, 3 percent of pregnancies).[8] The variety of services now provided by each level of nursery is presented in Table 1.

The drive for regionalization of perinatal care services represented a desire to decrease neonatal mortality and to improve the outcome for survivors. Several general principles guided the development of a regional perinatal care system. Regionalization of services was intended to improve accountability for the care of a specific population, provide a single standard of quality care, recognize differing care capabilities of institutions within a given geographical area, minimize patient movement (which increases risk), engender an optimal utilization of facilities and personnel, design care to serve special needs of different populations, and establish a structure that reflects the team character of perinatal care.[9]

During the 1970s, newborn and maternal care improved. Mortality during the neonatal period decreased. Social workers were brought onto the neonatal team in an effort to "humanize" care. Interest in the ethics of newborn medicine increased as questions were raised about what to do with severely defective or handicapped newborns who possibly might be kept alive.[10] By the 1980s, the state of the art has advanced to where nearly all modes of cardiopulmonary support and monitoring available for older patients are available for newborns.

Concern for the newborn now begins during pregnancy, involving a multidisciplinary effort. "The obstetrician becomes a fetal physiologist and continues his [or her] interest to include the postnatal state of the baby, while the neonatologist becomes the prenatal advocate and diagnostician of the fetus and watches over . . . [its] postnatal growth and development. The anesthesiologist is increasingly recognized as a valuable member of the team with his [or her] dual responsibility to ensure the comfort and safety of the mother, while safeguarding the integrity of the fetus and helping in the management of the newborn."[11] Add to this medical team the services of nurses, social workers, laboratory technicians, respiratory and pharmaceutical supports, and consulting

TABLE 1
Services Provided by Perinatal Facilities

Services	Level I	Level II	Level III
Complete prenatal care for maternity patient with no complications or with minor complications	X	X	X
Complete prenatal care for maternity patients with most complications		X	X
A special diagnostic and management clinic for high-risk prenatal patients			X
Risk identification scoring system	X	X	X
Management of uncomplicated labor and delivery of normal-term fetus	X	X	X
Prompt management of unexpected complications occurring during labor and delivery, including anesthesia, cesarean section, and blood administration		X	X
Management of complicated labor and delivery		X	X
Intrapartum intensive care			X
In-house anesthesia service		X	X
Electronic fetal monitoring	±	X	X
Physically separated facilities for obstetrics	X	X	X
Capability for resuscitation of depressed neonate at every delivery	X	X	X
Care for the healthy newborn	X	X	X
Stabilization and risk assessment of all neonates	X	X	X
Intravenous fluid administration to neonates	X	X	X
Management of most neonates who have complications up to short-term assisted ventilation		X	X
Continuous neonatal monitoring capability		X	X
Blood gases available on twenty-four-hour basis		X	X
Neonatal intensive care including assisted ventilation and hyperalimentation			X
Neonatal surgical capability			X
Availability of pediatric subspecialists in cardiology, genetics, and hematology			X
Care of mothers with no complications postpartum	X	X	X
Management of unexpected postpartum complications including hemorrhage and sepsis	X	X	X
Management of most postpartum complications		X	X
Data collection on performance and outcome	X	X	X
Laboratory services for electrolytes, bilirubin, blood glucose, calcium on twenty-four-hour basis	X	X	X
X-ray services with portable film capability on twenty-four-hour basis	X	X	X

Services	Level I	Level II	Level III
Laboratory services to assess fetal well-being and maturity		X	X
Diagnostic X-ray ultrasound		X	X
Nutritional consultation		X	X
Social service		X	X
Respiratory therapy consultation		X	X
Sterilization and family planning services	X	X	X
Follow-up developmental assessment clinic			X

medical and surgical specialists and the result is an extensive cadre of personnel and technology geared to maximize a newborn's chance to survive.

The focus on survival, or a decreased mortality rate, as a standard of success is reasonable when it is understood that a dissatisfaction with infant mortality rates was an incentive for the development of neonatology as a subspecialty. It is difficult, however, to determine with certainty the effect of newborn intensive care on declining mortality rates without randomized clinical trials. Other factors, such as lower rates of prematurity, improved maternal health, or improved maternal nutrition, may have a role. Nevertheless, by pooling mortality data from several neonatal intensive care units, Peter Budetti, a pediatrician at the University of California in San Francisco, and Peggy McManus, a researcher at the Institute for Health Policy Studies at the University of California in San Francisco, conclude "that neonatal medical care has played a significant role in bringing about the impressive reduction in infant mortality that has taken place in this country since 1965."[12] Further, in a different study, Budetti and associates determined that "it appears that the incidence of serious problems in survivors of neonatal intensive care is probably declining."[13] The mortality statistics since 1965 when major changes in perinatal[14] medical care began to take place indicate that neonatal deaths declined 35 percent between 1965 and 1975 compared to a 12 percent decline from 1950 to 1965.[15] Since 1970, nearly all— 88 percent—of the decline in infant mortality[16] has occurred in the neonatal period.[17] The mortality rate for the first twenty-eight days of life has declined steadily since 1930. The decline, however, has been most rapid between 1970 and 1980, the period of broad expansion of neonatal services.

The single most important factor in neonatal illness and mortality is birth weight. As an infant's birth weight goes down, its risk of death goes up. A second major indicator of neonatal death is gestational age. Like birth weight, the shorter the gestation before birth, the greater is the risk of death. Infants born between twenty and twenty-seven weeks of gestation have an eighty-times greater likelihood of death than infants born at term (forty weeks).[18] The third major type of problem for newborns is congenital anomalies, which account for nearly 20 percent of infant deaths.

It is in the first two prime areas of high risk—birth weight and gestational age—that neonatal care has been most visibly successful. Budetti and McManus report that since the advent of intensive care, the mortality rates for newborns weighing between 35 and 52½ ounces (1,001 and 1,500 grams) has declined from around 50 percent to less than 20 percent. For infants weighing less than 35 ounces (1,000 grams), mortality has declined from over 93 percent to about 50 percent.[19] Many low birth weight and premature infants who would have died before the development of neonatal intensive care are now surviving to lead normal lives. Others in this number who earlier would have died now survive but with abnormalities or neurological deficits. There is disagreement about the long-term impact of ventilatory support. Several studies show a higher incidence of neurodevelopmental, bronchopulmonary, and visual handicap in low birth weight infants receiving ventilation than for those not receiving ventilatory support.[20] Thus it is ironic that one of the interventions necessary to save life is linked to chronic problems that may limit a survivor's quality of life.

Data regarding the type and severity of morbidity or handicap experienced by some survivors are difficult to interpret. An extensive analysis sponsored by the Office of Technology Assessment of the United States Congress (OTA) reviewed reports from individual nurseries. The study revealed that "in general, the incidence of serious handicap is inversely proportional to birth weight. The most serious and frequent problems are reported in infants with very low birthweight, that is, less than 1500 grams."[21] Further, the OTA found that the percentage of low birth weight infants left with a serious impairment seems to have declined since the inception of intensive care.[22] This rather optimistic and supportive assessment may be of qualified value. As the authors confess, the data upon which their analyses are based were limited since much was drawn from reports of individual intensive care nurseries and their experience with in-born survivors, i.e., they were center-based rather than area-based studies. These findings are also limited by their coverage of a variety of different aspects of morbidity and use by their sources of different measurements of defect.[23]

Area-based analyses are believed to overcome patient selection biases that can skew the results of center-based studies. Several area-based studies have found that mortality rates for low (1000–1499 grams) and very low (500–999 grams) birth weight infants fell after the introduction of neonatal intensive care. But, these studies also found that the incidence of major handicaps among survivors did not change significantly, even though care became more sophisticated.[24]

Another burden, beyond an increased risk for illness related to neonatal care, is the financial cost. The cost of intensive and follow-up care for small, premature, or defective infants can have a devastating effect on a family's financial situation. For example, an early study found that the average cost to produce a "normal" survivor who weighed 35 ounces (1,000 grams) or less at birth was $88,058 (adjusted to September 1976 rates and *excluding* physicians' fees).[25] When the costs of survival for infants weighing less than 52½ ounces (approximately 1,499 grams) at birth are economically evaluated, given certain economic assumptions, it has been found that intensive care "represents a net drain on society's resources—that is, the program consumes more resources than it saves or creates."[26] The question that parents and society must answer is, How much are we willing to pay for survival and/or improved health outcomes?

Thus it appears that modern medical care for the newborn is able to save the lives of some infants who without these services would have much less chance to live. Fortunately for these survivors and for their care providers and society, many are expected to lead normal or near-normal lives without serious handicap. The financial cost of securing these results is not small. More attention to maternal and prenatal care might reduce the need for intensive neonatal care and, therefore, the financial cost of a normal survivor.

Apart from general concerns about rising costs of neonatal medical care and the uncertain long-term outcomes, the im-

proved survival data tend to be greeted enthusiastically. The reaction to those infants who survive with severe physical or mental
handicap has been mixed based on concerns about the quality of
life for the survivor and the impact of the infant on family and
social resources. These cases generate medical and moral debate
about the adequacy of survival alone as the primary objective and
standard of success for neonatology. To acknowledge quality of
life as an equally important objective and standard for the treatment of newborns entails a recognition that something beyond
mere living makes existence good. A neonatologist expressed
concern for these infants in stark terms: "What gives me the right
to save this baby so that mother can wheel it around in a wagon
and bring it back to the clinic?" In addition to worries about
whether life is truly in the interest of certain infants who will survive with severe deficits or deformities, increased consideration
is being given to the effect their survival will have on family and
society. Judgments are being made by physicians and parents in
consultation that when there is no prospect for meaningful existence medical efforts to prolong life are not warranted. Selected
infants are not treated.[27] Their deaths are anticipated, even desired. All things considered, their interest, in isolation and in relation to others, is determined not to require medical support.

A Context for Intersecting Interests

When one observes the way in which decisions about imperiled
newborns are made over a period of time, the nature of the moral
community as a pluralism is displayed. The identification and
rank-ordering of competing interests seem never to be identical
from one case to another. The general interests of infant, family,
health personnel, and society are acknowledged but refracted
through the particular circumstances of each case. Neonatologists
are placed in a delicate position of participating in the process of
making decisions, taking account of the multiple interests in conflict, and struggling with parents to discern a morally right course.
These sorts of decisions, when approached conscientiously, impose a grave burden of responsibility on the principals to explore
options, consider possible consequences, and give due regard to
the interests of everyone concerned. In the case that follows, I

analyze and illustrate how the interests of these several parties may conflict and influence decisions for or against treatment.

A twenty-eight-year-old woman in her sixth pregnancy gave birth to a 70-ounce (2,000-gram) male infant at the thirty-fourth week of gestation. Two earlier pregnancies resulted in stillbirths. Three children under age ten were at home. The family was indigent. At birth the baby made no respiratory effort, was blue and floppy. He was ventilated in the delivery room and transported to neonatal intensive care. Numerous diagnostic tests were performed. The baby was found to have a muscle enzyme deficiency (myophosphorylase deficiency), a condition for which no therapy exists. This diagnosis was difficult to make. Consultants from several subspecialties examined the infant. The notes on the baby's chart read like a detective story. The physicians were intrigued and excited in their pursuit of a mysterious condition.

Four pediatric neurologists were part of the investigative team. Three of these consultants and the neonatologists agreed with the diagnosis, one neurologist did not. Additional tests were requested. Conversations took place with neurologists in other cities. The conviction of the dissenting neurologist was that there was a possibility of another diagnosis, one whose prognosis was better. While another diagnosis was being explored, novel therapies were advocated in an effort to prove an alternate diagnosis or to observe the natural course of this rare disease if the original diagnosis was shown ultimately to be accurate.

The parents were advised of the diagnosis and prognosis, as well as of the conflict between consultants, in a meeting of parents, neonatologists, and chaplain. They were told that the baby's muscles had no strength, including the muscles necessary for breathing. The prospects for a change were minimal or nonexistent. They were told that the baby had an increased risk for infection and aspiration, could not suck or swallow, and probably would develop contractures. They could see the baby's muscles wasting away. Observing this deterioration was painful to them. They considered the situation of the baby and instructed the neonatologists to keep supporting their baby if there was hope for his recovery. But if there was no hope for near-normal survival, they did not want anything else done diagnostically that would increase the baby's pain only to satisfy the curiosity of the physicians and increase their financial obligation to the hospital.

Four days later, and after continued efforts by the single neurological consultant to establish an alternate diagnosis, another
conference with the parents took place. As before they expressed
concern for the pain and suffering of their baby. If the baby would
be paralyzed or a pulmonary cripple they did not want heroic
efforts undertaken, including resuscitation or other interventions.
After another four days, and the continued manipulation of the
infant, the father became much more assertive and protective of
the baby. He specifically refused all but comforting interventions
for his baby. He would not agree to an autopsy, which he saw as
a self-interested request by the dissenting neurologist. The father
said that he felt manipulated by the dissenting consultant whose
ego and curiosity, in his judgment, were being satisfied at the
expense of his baby's comfort. As before, now for the third time,
he requested that the inevitable death of the baby not be prolonged. He did not consider a slow, drawn-out death in the interest of the baby or the family.

The dissenting neurologist persisted in the struggle with the
neonatologists and other consultants to accept a different diagnosis more therapeutically approachable. The father, exasper-
ated, threatened to take the child home, knowing that it could
not breathe without the respirator. The neurologist, when advised of the father's threat, wrote in the chart. ''I don't believe
anyone, even a father, has a right to decide for the death of a
baby. This case should be discussed with the District Attorney
before treatment is stopped.'' Following this entry, the debate between the physicians grew more intense in chart notes. Literature
and authorities were referenced. Each side was unconvinced by
the other. In the interim, the baby continued to waste away. The
parents felt overwhelmed by the intransigence of the consultant.
They considered the situation out of their hands, now the twenty-
third day of the baby's life. Finally, one week later, as the medical
standoff continued, the baby died of cardiac arrest. Resuscitative
efforts failed.

From my perspective, this was a distressing case involving
conflicting interests. Before the inception of intensive care technologies this baby would have died soon after birth. Had the respirator been disconnected the baby would have died before it
did in the hospital. Given a fatal diagnosis and the absence of
therapeutic capability, the interests generally imputed to infants
of life, health, and quality of existence were impossible to realize.

The only interest the infant could be said to have was that of an easy death. The family expressed the baby's interests in terms of wanting him to survive but not wanting life to be a burden to him. The protective posture that they attempted was intended by them to advance the baby's interests as they understood them. The emotional and financial burden this infant's survival and subsequent care would have imposed on the parents and other children were secondary for the parents to the child's interest in an easy death. The family was indigent, dependent on governmental assistance for the basics of life. They were accustomed to adversity. Two children had been stillborn. Being out of work was routine. Medical care in public clinics was all they knew. The parents felt that one more burden, if the baby lived, did not pose a great threat to the limited opportunity that they had to pursue goals.

The intense disagreement among the physicians and between one consultant and the parents and all other physicians created an impasse that compounded the pain and suffering of everyone involved. The personal bias of the dissenting neurologist became clear in the chart note objecting to a withdrawal of support. The extent to which personal interest or bias influenced professional opinion is subject only to speculation. The dispute between the dissenter and all others (neonatologists, consultants, and parents) reflected differing interpretations of diagnostic data, as well as differing assessments of interests and duties related to those interpretations. While the respective conflicting interests and desires were being negotiated the infant's life was supported. Invasive diagnostic, monitoring, and supportive interventions continued. The baby's body and life shrank before their eyes while costs mounted.

Hospital and physician charges are a matter of societal interest in this case. The parents were not able to pay these expenses. Medicaid was the responsible entity. Because Medicaid is a governmentally funded program, society's interest was involved in the financial allocation of resources. Its interest was symbolic to the extent that the decent care of this infant during its dying reflected our concern for one another. It is difficult to see how the state's interest to protect life could be furthered since the baby's disease was fatal. The suggestion of the dissident neurologist to consult with the district attorney had the potential to involve the state directly in the decision-making process. But assuming the accuracy of the terminal diagnosis, nothing that a court could order would have altered the outcome of this case except for an authorization to discontinue life support, which would have meant an earlier death for the infant and less suffering for all others.

Since an infant cannot express wishes, others necessarily act in its behalf. Articulating the infant's interests and balancing them with competing interests of others can be agonizing to those who bear the responsibility to so act. Neonatologists frequently are in a bind. Ideally committed to the care of the newborn, sensitive to the situation of the infant's family, and cognizant of the state's interests, they are at the center of conflict, expected somehow to possess sufficient moral wisdom to choose and act rightly. In addition, they are expected not to manipulate all of the parties to these tragedies in order to enhance their own professional, financial, or personal interests.

A Sustaining Presence

There have been numerous efforts to express in an image or model the role a physician has in his or her ministrations to sick or dying individuals.[28] These images bring to life, personalize, and communicate perceptions and expectations about the role of a physician in clinical encounters.[29] It should be emphasized, however, that models do not provide answers for particular moral questions in medicine in general and neonatology in particular. This would require models to do the work of ethics, i.e., moral analysis. Answers to moral questions, in medicine or elsewhere, are based in moral theory. Moral principles, rules, values, and ideals shape answers, not models that portray the dynamic, interpersonal character of therapeutic relationships.

The physician has been viewed as a technician, priest, colleague, parent, fighter, teacher, contractor, and covenanter. Each model captures something of what physicians represent and do. The images of contractor and covenanter have been proposed as inclusive images that acknowledge other images as subsidiary ones that help to illuminate important aspects of the physician's role. Subordinate images are seen to enrich the inclusive metaphor by giving it greater specificity in practice. The comprehensive and subordinate metaphors are seen to support one another in a coherent pattern. Together they shed light on the nature of the physician's role and the character of the relationship of which he or she is a key part.[30]

I have no fundamental quarrel with or objection to the images of contract and covenant as they have been described.[31] Each is an effort to say something constructive about the moral terms of the relationship between patient and physician. However, another metaphor might be able to avoid a potential complaint against each. Contract might be criticized for being too commercial in tone for an intimate, human relationship. Covenant might be criticized for being too religious in tone for a secular, professional encounter. As an alternate metaphor that escapes these two complaints, I propose that the physician, or more particularly the neonatologist, be seen as a sustaining presence.

The metaphor of a sustaining presence incorporates the thrusts or emphases of the previously mentioned models: concerns for technical competence (technician); awareness of the value-ladened nature of the medical event (priest); shared objectives as a basis for relationship (colleague); intent to struggle against what can be defeated (fighter); instructive about the nature of the human condition (teacher); behavior that is protective and nurturing (parent); responsive and dynamic but limited by the rights and liberties of the parties (covenanter and contractor). The contribution of the image of sustaining presence, however, is not in its ability to accommodate the themes of its competitors. Rather it is in its ability to represent the unique circumstances and associated requirements of individual cases. In order to illustrate this claim more needs to be said about clinical relationships in general.[32]

The relationship between adult patients and physicians is taking increasingly divergent forms in the pursuit of multiple objectives. For example, an obstetrician can help a patient control her reproductive function by aborting her pregnancy. The next patient may be helped in her quest to become pregnant by performing artificial insemination or attempting in vitro fertilization with embryo implant: same obstetrician, one profession of medicine, two patients with differing requests that reflect their respective notions of what is good for them at a particular time. Physicians are rarely able or desirous of assuming full control of their patients, at least in the sense that control entails an imposition on the patient of the end to be sought and the means by which it is to be pursued. An authoritarianism representative of extreme medical paternalism is steadily yielding to a negotiated relationship and a shared responsibility by the parties for what takes place. The notion that there is only one proper or moral course determined by a benevolent physician has given way in an enlightened, pluralistic environment to an acceptance of many possibly proper means and ends in which the physician's benevolence as the sole motive and standard of service is less important. The zone of discretionary judgment of physicians is being narrowed by the injunctions of moral and legal rules, and greater participation by patients in the design of their health care. It is argued in this volume that in newborn medicine, the voice of the patient in most instances is that of the parent. The responsibility borne by adult patients rests upon parents in neonatology. It is they, in their fiduciary role, who are presumed to have the requisite competence, skills, and ability to make the intricate assessments necessary to make decisions on behalf of an infant and for the family.

It is possible only to stipulate in a general way that patient-physician relationships are established to seek cure where possible and the least evil otherwise.[33] But in addition to these formal objectives, the relationship materially is a context in which care and concern for the misfortune of another are expressed. It is occasioned by the sickness, pain, suffering, or threat of death that another experiences. The nature of the human condition as vulnerable is a fact that we tend to deny. Pregnancies are started with the hope that the risks to fetus and mother will never be made manifest. And when that which is feared becomes a reality in the form of severe disease or defect in the newborn we turn to medicine to reverse the destructive process and to erect barriers between the newborn and death or severe disability. We admire and support those who protect us from death and the negative effects of its appearances.

When misfortune attends the birth of a baby, parents turn to neonatologists whose represented powers are hoped to engender health for the infant. The loss of parental power in sickness to protect and nurture is compensated for by the powers of the neonatal team to whom parents turn for help. The neonatal team symbolizes relief and protection. The consultation and the subsequent process is a joint venture wherein resources are marshalled to defeat the threat, learn to live with the limitations it imposes, or to accept its realization. When parents are excluded from the decisional process their sense of impotence may be increased. Those basic acts of parenting that help to secure a bond with an infant may be denied with both parent and infant suffering the consequences in the future. These critical moments can be seized as opportunities to learn about life and death, to learn early that parenting entails a responsibility to make hard decisions that are of the life and death variety.[34]

Parents usually suffer during these periods of uncertainty and danger. Neonatologists can help to relieve this suffering by imparting meaning to a situation in which meaninglessness seems the only explanation.[35] The reverse also is possible. Parents may help neonatologists to discover meaning in what otherwise appears senseless. How this is done for particular cases cannot be specified in advance. On the one hand, much depends on the condition of the infant, the social, economic, religious, moral, and educational background of the parents and, on the other hand, on a similar variety of factors for neonatologists. Performing well in this aspect of patient care may require of neonatologists and the entire neonatal team greater energy and creativity than performing well in physical diagnosis and treatment.

To parents who suffer, the presence of neonatologists can provide assurance that they and their threatened newborn are not excluded from the human community in which care and concern is mediated. In the experience of sickness and suffering the weak (infant) and strong (parents and neonatal team) are bound together in a sustaining alliance. Rather than being abandoned, the sick and suffering parties in these tragic circumstances are a central concern. Life-prolonging efforts may be seen as a means to affirm the value placed on human life. Alternately, if an infant is allowed to die or assisted in dying, this too may be seen as a means of affirming those cherished powers that give life meaning but are believed never possible for the infant to develop. The infant/parent-neonatologist relationship is a joint endeavor in pursuit of identifiable goods and the avoidance of identifiable evils. It is a relation initiated in a situation of threat and agony. It is a relation generated by a situation of uncertainty and potential danger.

The parent-neonatologist relationship necessarily deals with uncertainty, and the uncertainty within clinical medicine is far-reaching. Yet physicians tend not to disclose their doubts, perhaps in order to prompt compliance with their recommendations and to maintain the esteem of peers. This reluctance to expose one's doubts is consistent with those images of physicians that symbolize strength, superiority, or power: healer, teacher, fighter, parent, technician, and priest. These images suggest that the physician's duties are defined in terms of and derived from his or her strength. But when the neonatologist's technical strength is useless or its exercise may not be wise in light of longer term consequences, his or her duties to parents and newborn do not cease. A better image of neonatologists, and for all medical clinicians, is that of a sustaining presence. This image allows for strength and weakness in the clinician. It does not imply that the neonatologist's duties are tied to strength alone. It suggests that embodied weakness can be present to a weakened body in a preserving and affirming manner. It calls attention to the value of fidelity in the presence of uncertainty and degeneration. An image of sustaining presence can represent the neonatologist's duties in cases where cure is possible and where it is not. It does not suggest expectations of the neonatal team that are impossible or unreasonable. It allows for fallibility and doubt.

Neonatologists can provide parents with few guarantees. They can promise parents to be available to them and their child, and to sustain all in technological and personal ways, and to the degrees possible and warranted. The neonatal team can join with parents in a journey into a dangerous unknown. Each assumes some risks through and some responsibility for the process and its conclusion. The alliance is one of relative strength and weakness. Their task is to negotiate a reality that includes pain, suffering, sickness, perhaps handicap or death. The infant/parent-neonatologist relationship is one in which the participants embrace life as it is and attempt to achieve whatever good is possible, perhaps in the presence of the inevitable. The unthinkable may become actual and life with no prospect of meaning, or death, may come. Efforts to help may fail or even harm the intended beneficiary. Finitude may be reluctantly accepted.

The parent-neonatologist relationship becomes a context not only of intersecting interests but also one in which something of the nature of the human condition is learned. Each participant learns that these unfortunate situations are vignettes of life, that life is vulnerable, and that what was conceived in hope can result in despair. In these situations, a sustaining presence can teach parents the wisdom of nature. Some newborns can be helped by medicine to make the transition from womb to world. Others are unable to live, nature has not equipped them sufficiently. Even with medical help, they cannot make the transformation from fetus to person. As a sustaining presence, physicians teach parents about nature's workings, diagnosis, prognosis, and therapeutic options, if any. Parents, already confronted with the risks of reproduction, are then responsible for defining what is important within life, recognize what dangers exist, decide what certain goods are worth, and perhaps end up choosing among evils.

In these tragic situations, the sustaining presence of neonatologists can powerfully state that the infant and parents are valued by others. Out of this affirmation the parents may be better able to exercise the burden of making decisions regarding the care of their infant. The integrity with which they do so can be enhanced by the presence of honest, loyal, and helping neonatologists. Being a sustaining presence does not sanction an imposition of the neonatologist's values upon parents who hold different but equally sustainable moral commitments and values. Thus, the sharing between neonatologist and parent in making treatment decisions does not consist in imposing upon either the requirements of the other. In short, the moral integrity of all is respected. No party should be coerced to accept a decision or participate in an action that is contrary to a personal moral norm or outside professional or social limits of tolerance. The relationship between parent and neonatologist consists of a shared negotiation with tragic circumstances.[36] In the role of sustaining presence, neonatologists share responsibility with parents for the process and the results. But neither bears the burden alone. Neonatologists ought not to tell parents which morally permissible option to choose. This may mean that some parents will choose life and others will accept death for their severely impaired newborn. Either course holds potential for good and grief.

A metaphor of the neonatologist as a sustaining presence seems appropriate for health care in the setting of a moral pluralism. As a sustaining presence, neonatologists may join and cooperate with parents in determining the baby's and family's collective best interest. Each party, parent and neonatologist, sustains the other by a constant affirmation of the moral and nonmoral goods of life and relationship expressed in a context of care and concern. Neonatologists are not bound, according to this image of their role, to any single moral vision that prescribes only one end and accepts only those means that contribute to that end.

As a sustaining presence and within limits imposed by personal conscience, professional ethics, or legal restraints, neonatal medicine can serve a variety of interests that reflect diverse moral visions as they relate to the medical care of defective newborn infants.

Priority of Parental Authority

The cooperative and consultative role for neonatologists that I have described as a "sustaining presence" is radically different from a more decisive and authoritarian role advocated by other commentators on the ethics of neonatology. Some would place the responsibility for making treatment decisions on physicians. Still others support committees, courts, or some combination or sequence of these as more appropriate deciders than parents. The reasons why these other candidates are favored have been nicely summarized in a very fine survey of literature on the ethics of neonatology by Robert Weir,[37] an ethicist at Oklahoma State University.

Some consider neonatologists the preferred decision makers because of their role and specialized knowledge. They argue that neonatologists are more distant and less affected by the stress and grief that accompany the birth of a defective newborn. As a result, they are able to be more objective than parents in determining the baby's best interests. They are also better positioned, because of their greater knowledge of and experience with defective newborns, to make informed and rational decisions regarding treatment. Finally, it is argued that neonatologists can be consistent in their decisions. By being involved with more than one instance of a particular defect, disease, or impairment, they are able to treat similar cases similarly, thereby escaping charges of discrimination and injustice. These arguments, however, are not persuasive.

Diagnoses can be mistaken and the severity of handicaps are better stated as probabilities. When the best available medical data are gathered, neonatologists, as such, are no better qualified to make decisions that are essentially moral in nature than any other possible decision maker. Weir objects to the claim of objectivity for two reasons. In my opinion, the first seems mistaken and the second does not go far enough. He thinks "pediatric specialists have a serious bias in favor of normal, healthy children. Having cared for numerous handicapped infants and observed problems that confront such infants, pediatricians often are inclined to view anomalous newborns as living tragedies that should have been terminated prior to birth."[38] If this refers to pediatric specialists other than neonatologists then I am inclined to agree. But, in my experience, neonatologists, who do not personally follow graduates of the intensive care unit throughout childhood, tend to minimize the negative possibilities for the infant and family. After neonatologists work their magic the baby goes home. The infant's health care becomes the responsibility of other pediatricians. Care of the family falls to clergy, social workers, psychiatrists, pediatricians, and the family's other physicians. The neonatologists who enabled a tragedy to be perpetuated often remain detached and unaffected.

A second potential conflict of interest is a neonatologist's bias toward research and experimentation. "Rather than trying to assess treatment options in terms of the best interests of individual neonatal patients, they tend to view patients—especially those with the most serious, possibly exotic conditions—as relatively rare opportunities to advance the cause of neonatal medicine as a science."[39] This criticism does not go far enough. Professional egos and personal values can also distort the neonatologist's assessment of the baby's interests. Further, it should be observed that much of neonatal medicine is research and experimentation—it is an "infant" subspecialty that utilizes innovative procedures in the hope of acceptable results and standardization. In short, neonatologists often undertake novel, creative interventions in a good faith effort to do what they reasonably can to save the life of a neonate or minimize the negative effects of its disease or defect. Finally, the argument for consistency is qualified by the observation that external pressures can influence decisions about classes of patients or individual patients. Changes in the law or its enforcement can cause neonatologists to treat diagnoses that previously would have gone untreated. Similarly, assertive parents may cause neonatologists to comply with parental wishes, either to save or let die, in cases where the treatment decision would have been different without parental intervention.

Hospital committees are touted by some as a better alternative to parents or physicians as proxies for neonates. They have the advantage of having a multidisciplinary membership, providing a broader expertise for dealing with difficult cases. A committee can provide a neutral forum in which conflicts regarding treatment can be adjudicated. It can serve as a check on parents and physicians who agree to act against a neonate's perceived best interests. Lastly, if a committee member is a trained ethicist there may be a greater likelihood that moral principles and rules will be applied consistently from case to case.

There are several problems with the committee option, especially if its role is more than advisory. One is that decisions may need to be made quickly and it may be difficult to convene a meeting on short notice. Another is that the member with the relevant expertise may not be in attendance. Then, once in session, there are no guarantees that the committee will function efficiently, fairly, or effectively. A final problem is that any committee, whether advisory or authorized to decide, tends to reduce parental autonomy and physician discretion. Advocates of the authority of parents or physicians to decide, therefore, object to committees as usurping another's rightful role. Another complaint is that a committee's distance from a case, its insulation from the short- and long-term consequences of its decision, is a strong argument in favor of vesting decision-making authority in those individuals most intimately connected to the baby.[40] A final criticism is the committee's potential to substitute and enforce, if given the authority to decide, its collective values, which may be no more or less worthy than those of the parents or physicians. Apart from factual considerations (diagnosis, prognosis, therapy) for which committees can effect checks and balances, they do not seem to improve the likelihood that "better" treatment decisions will be made.

The third proposed alternative to parental authority is the courts. Calls for courts to be primary decision makers appear based on a disputable presumption that the best decision maker is one who is a disinterested party. Advocates of the courts argue that only in this forum can a baby's best interests be protected. A judge can gather the relevant facts and consider the interests of all relevant parties, including the neonate whose needs and claims are represented by a guardian *ad litem*. It can be said in response that courts in practice are subject to the same objections voiced against hospital committees. They reduce parent autonomy, hinder medical discretion, can be slow, inconsistent, and unaffected. Finally, judges as individuals are subject to issuing opinions based as much or more on personal values as on the law.

Robert Weir is not satisfied to grant absolute authority to decide to any single proxy—physician, committee, court, or parent. He favors a best-interest standard for decision making regarding anomalous newborns. This standard requires that decisions be made on the basis of "whether the medical procedure will on balance benefit or harm the incompetent person."[41] The interests of the neonate take precedence over any and all competing interests according to this standard of judgment. Further, best interest is understood as what "most reasonable persons would choose in a particular situation of moral choice."[42]

Having settled on the best interests of the neonate as the primary standard and sole end of decision making, Weir adopts a "serial or sequential ordering of decision makers . . . for determining the best interests of neonatal patients"[43] that was proposed by James Childress,[44] an ethicist at the University of Virginia. A procedure that can involve all of the suggested proxies is seen to offer greater protection of the neonate's best interests, allow for appeals to a higher proxy in the serial ordering, and permit decisions of a lower proxy to be contravened when indicated.

The Childress-Weir serial ordering places parents of defective newborns as primary decision makers, but their right to decide can be overridden in at least three circumstances: "when they simply cannot understand the relevant medical facts of a case, when they are emotionally unstable, and when they appear to put their own interests before those of the defective newborn."[45] Weir comments; "[N]o birth-defective newborn should be left to die untreated merely because of the desires or discretion of parents, especially when there appears to be a conflict of interest between the parents and the child."[46] Physicians should be empowered, according to Weir, to override parents because of their superior knowledge, experience, and disinterested role. In doing so, neonatologists become patient advocates who, on their own authority, in certain circumstances, act contrary to parental direction, or "in borderline cases" turn to an intensive care committee for counsel. The authority of neonatologists, in Weir's scheme, is limited or checked when the interests pursued are other than the best interests of the neonate, e.g., a neonatologist's research, financial, or turf interests.

The neonatal intensive care committee is the center piece of serial decision making. The committee is the "court of appeals," the in-house locus for mediation of disputes between parents and the neonatal team. It oversees decisions agreed upon by parents and neonatologists to assure that the infant's best interests are being served. In its advisory role, the NICU committee constitutes a procedural safeguard against the abuse of a neonate's interests. Courts are a last resort. Weir prefers that decisions be made and disputes resolved without judicial review. However, there may be rare instances in which, on following a report by a nurse or social worker, a judge concludes that the best interests of an infant are not served by the decisions of the first three proxies (parent, neonatologist, committee). If a judge finds that the parents and physicians are not acting in the best interests of the newborn, custody of the baby could be taken from the parents and criminal proceedings against the physicians and/or parents could follow. Weir doubts that courts would have to take this sort of action very often in cases involving institutions with well-balanced, effectively working neonatal intensive care committees.

While I can appreciate the benevolent and protective intent of a formal serial decision-making process, it is not, in my opinion, able to withstand certain criticisms. As a result, it is not a significant improvement over relying generally on parental judgments. As stated, Weir feels that neonatologists should be able to override parents who do not comprehend the facts, are emotionally unstable, or who do not give the neonate's interests priority. Comprehension and competency are conditions for making all treatment decisions; the notion of informed consent makes sense only if this is so.[47] We are not told by Weir what level of parental incomprehension, or what type or degree of parental emotional instability, is sufficient for neonatologists to assume decisional authority. Such a vague standard is no standard. If a neonatologist agrees with a parental decision, comprehension and emotional state appear irrelevant. If a neonatologist disagrees, parental comprehension and emotional state become issues, and bases for overriding.[48]

Finally, there are no compelling reasons why a severely *defective* newborn's interests should take priority over those of parents or siblings. Because an imperiled newborn is either defective, young, innocent, or weak, in and of itself, is not a sufficient reason to require other moral agents to sacrifice legitimate interests.

Justice requires that the interest or due of each party materially affected by a decision to prolong the life of a defective newborn or to accept its death warrants consideration. The newborn's interest is one among others, each having a prima facie claim to recognition and advancement. Decision makers in situations of conflict are responsible for weighing the respective interests of the relevant parties, to order and choose among them on the basis of morally licit criteria. Simply because one set of interests are attached to a newborn human is not a sufficient reason to give it priority over the interests of others. Nevertheless, an imperiled infant is an object of compassionate care because he or she is valued in its present state, not for what it may never become.

Giving neonatologists the trump card or empowering them to override parental judgments regarding treatment for severely defective newborns seems mainly to authorize a substitution of the physician's values for the parent's values. Only in those instances in which parental judgments go beyond the reasonable limits accepted by the moral community, in which parents are absent or incompetent, or in which unforeseen events require decisions not previously guided by parents, are neonatologists justified in assuming parental authority.

In situations of conflict between parents and neonatal medical personnel that cannot be resolved by good faith negotiation, an appeal to the courts, rather than in-house committees, appears in order. Committees can attempt to mediate a dispute, but they have no authority to settle an argument. In an impasse, only courts have authority to rule. The proposed advantages of the committee system turn on the idea that decision making must aim primarily at realizing the best interests of a severely defective or diseased newborn whose life is in jeopardy. The primacy of the interests of this sort of newborn, in my opinion, has not been convincingly shown. Further, if parents and neonatologists have arrived at their respective positions after a full and careful consideration of the issues and interests involved, the capacity of a committee to move either party seems questionable.

Judicial review is aptly described as a last resort. No one really wins in these situations. Once again, as with committee review, the best interests of the neonate are asserted by Weir as primary. Yet in these borderline cases, best interests tend to be reflections of individual moral and nonmoral values. Though a judge's opinion may be couched in legal terms, it may not be necessarily a better or more compelling decision from a point of view that embraces a moral pluralism. Though I am sympathetic with the respective concerns that are expressed by locating decision-making authority in courts, committees, or physicians, I am not convinced that the supposed advantages substituting any or all of them for parents in the great majority of cases is warranted, all things considered.

Advocates of parental authority tend to do so out of regard for parental autonomy.[49] Proponents argue that a restriction of parental discretion in these situations is arbitrary. Parents are generally free to decide the type of education, religious and moral training, and most medical interventions for their children. Assigning responsibility for decisions to others during the neonatal period seems inconsistent and unnecessary. The emotional bonds formed for the newborn during pregnancy are believed to persist after birth, even though the resulting baby is not the one the parents had anticipated. This commitment to the newborn, though perhaps distorted by the birth of a defective or diseased baby, is believed still to be biased toward the continued life of the baby, not its death. Finally, it is argued that parents and immediate families will experience most closely the respective benefits and losses of the baby's continued life or death. As such, parents properly should decide for or against treatment.[50]

Some ethicists, physicians, and lay people are troubled by the prospect of relying exclusively on parents for these sorts of decisions. For example, Weir questions the competency of parents who may be "emotionally devastated," "inadequately informed," "virtually ignorant of alternatives," or "unable to understand" the current situation and/or implications of their baby's condition. The second and third potential weaknesses would not appear to be the parents' fault. If they are inadequately informed and/or ignorant of their alternatives, it seems the blame should be placed on professionals responsible for communicating this information and options to them. Parents, like everyone in every circumstance, decide on the basis of the data they have, whether the decision involves the purchase of an automobile or the nontreatment of a defective or diseased newborn. Similarly, parents said to be "unable to understand" may not have been told the relevant information in language and ways within their comprehension.

An assertion of their failure to understand can easily camouflage a preference to deprive parents of information and decisions that are rightfully theirs. Parents who truly cannot understand, despite the best efforts of others, would appear incompetent to make any decision regarding their children, not just treatment decisions for a defective newborn. If so, custody should be removed from them because of their incompetency, not because of the condition of the newborn. Lastly, "emotional devastation" is a slippery criterion. Does Weir refer to psychotic reactions or to ordinary grief? What degree and type of parental reaction is sufficient to remove from them decisional authority? We are not told. Babies for whom life or death is genuinely a choice usually can be stabilized in order to buy the time necessary for parents to regain composure and make considered judgments regarding the continuation or cessation of certain interventions.

Weir's objections to parents continues: "[I]t is a false assumption to think that all parents in these circumstances have the capacity to be either altruistic or impartial toward the handicapped newborns in their families. . . . In promoting their own psychological and financial interests, or protecting their chosen life-style and possibly other children at home, some parents simply cannot make impartial judgments about whether a defective newborn should receive treatment or die untreated."[51] In response, altruists may deserve our esteem, but absolute selflessness is beyond common understandings of moral duty. Impartiality is required by the canons of justice in situations of choice in which the parties chosen among are alike in morally relevant ways. It has not been shown, however, that severely defective or diseased newborns are sufficiently like other members of the moral community in relevant ways such as to require equal regard or impartiality.

Weir's final worry reflects his desire for consistent decisions based on moral principles and criteria "generally acceptable to other persons." He fears that if parents are given an "absolute right" to decide "there exists virtually no possibility for consistency from case to case." Some babies will live or die on the basis of parental determinations of the infant's best interests, others on the basis of "parental inclination, bias, whim, or whatever," and still others on the basis of the abilities of neonatologists to persuade parents.[52] I could not agree more with Weir's preference for decisions to be made in the light of relevant moral principles, rules, and values. However, as attractive as consistency is, the circumstances of particular cases usually are such that they are rarely, if ever, identical in morally relevant ways. This means that the interests of neonates and relevant others necessarily and appropriately will vary from case to case.

The potential for neonatologists to persuade parents to follow a preferred course ought not to be underestimated. Not only is this a corruption of the professional role and authority, it manipulates parents, robs them of their autonomy, and denies them an opportunity to face head-on the responsibilities of parenthood. Making life less difficult for someone (i.e., parents of defective or diseased newborns) by relieving them of the anxiety of making a hard decision may not be an appropriate way to express care and concern for them. No doubt there is a danger that treatment decisions may not be carefully reasoned morally, but this danger is not limited to parents. For example, a resident in neonatology who has been without sleep for hours, or who has fought with his or her superior, or who is fatigued by responding to the multiple problems of a baby that does not get better is as likely to give short shrift to carefully reasoned moral rules and principles in making a life or death decision.

In short, neonatologists are to advise and cooperate, according to the arguments provided above, with parents who are responsible for deciding the fate of their imperiled newborn. Committees may offer consultation services to parents and/or medical personnel. They ought not, however, have authority to make these decisions. Courts already have authority to decide, but they ought not do so unless the parents are absent or disqualified. In my experience, parents almost without exception endeavor to make good decisions based upon a fair evaluation of the intersecting interests of all concerned. Their judgments tend to be reasoned and reasonable, some for treatment and others against treatment, only rarely going beyond the limits of reason that a morally pluralistic society would find acceptable. Even though there may be instances of unreasonable judgments by parents that warrant contravention, it appears to me, all things considered, that the burden of proof rests on those who would depart from the custom of granting parents the prima facie right and responsibility to make the treatment decisions for severely defective or diseased newborns.

5

Making Treatment Decisions

THE CASE REPORTS provided in earlier chapters point out some of the factors that influence decisions for treatment or nontreatment of impaired newborns. There is a maxim in medicine that no two cases are ever alike. Though cases may be similar, the uniqueness of each case stems not only from the disease but also from nonmedical factors particular to each patient. The factors that are given priority in deciding individual cases reflect an understanding of the medical situation as well as its assessment in light of, at least in part, the decider's moral and value commitments. This chapter analyzes two approaches to a determination of what is morally required or allowed under adverse circumstances. In addition, proposals regarding the process of making decisions will be made.

Moral Status of Newborn Humans

One approach to determining the nature and degree of one's moral obligation to a severely diseased or deformed newborn is based on the *status* of that newborn as a person or nonperson. This standard is commonly used in other areas of life. For example, household insects are considered pests. Roaches and ants are not perceived to be persons with inalienable rights to life or rights to eat from the family pantry. Their extermination is not seen as a moral wrong. They are not even considered objects of compassion, that is to say, they may be killed violently (swatting) without offending the moral sensitivities of the community.

Household pets are a different matter. Dogs and cats are seen as companions or friends. Woofer and Kitty are not usually considered to have the rights of persons but nevertheless are objects of our compassion. Torturing or starving them is considered indecent at best and, perhaps, morally wrong at worst. Pets tend to be valued more highly than insects but less highly than normal human children and adults. Killing a dog or cat may upset lovers of pets, but it is not restrained unless animal cruelty laws are broken. Thus, it appears, at least intuitively and in practice, that pet dogs and cats have a status in the community that warrants humane treatment but not necessarily a right to life.

Our intuitions about these matters are more revealing when we consider creatures who have the same capacities as normal adults but who are not human. Millions of people saw the movie *E.T.*, which told the story of an extraterrestrial creature abandoned on earth. If my perception of the audience's reaction is correct, viewers felt that E.T. had a right not to be killed and a right to be sustained. When he died as a result of the action of government agents, there was a sense that E.T. had been wronged, not just treated inhumanely or indecently. E.T. was perceived to have a moral status equivalent to normal adult humans. In short, E.T. was considered as much of a person as the adult humans who pursued him and the children who befriended him.

These several illustrations show that people do, in fact, classify creatures within or without the community of persons. By so doing, some creatures are afforded protection and support and others are not. The issue to be explored in this section is the moral status of human newborns. In particular, we are concerned to discover if a severely impaired neonate, or a neonate with a disvalued prognosis, is subject to the same protection and/or support provided to healthy newborns, older children, or adults.

Consider three cases. Case A: A pregnant woman was found by ultrasound examination to be carrying two fetuses. Unfortunately, one fetus did not move and was believed to have died in utero. The pregnancy was continued until thirty weeks at which time a ceasarean section delivery was performed. Twin A was born with no problems other than those routinely associated with prematurity. Twin B was born alive, not dead as was suspected from the ultrasound exam. However, it is difficult to be certain about what to call this second product of conception. Twin B was alive but did not bear any resemblance to a human fetus. There were no limbs, head, or differentiated internal organs. The mass of tissue was alive, profused by an umbilical cord that was joined to the umbilicus of Twin A. Obviously, when the umbilical cord was severed the tissue died. How should this mass of tissue be described? Did it have a right to live? Were the physicians obligated to attempt to sustain its life? Were birth and death certificates necessary?

Case B: A 6-pound male infant was born to a young unwed mother. The newborn was normal in all respects except for obvious extensive absences of skin over the forearms, hands, legs, and feet. In addition, large blisters were observed on the buttocks. The baby was taken to the neonatal intensive care unit where a diagnosis of epidermolysis bullosa dystrophica was made. This disease is similar in appearance to third-degree burns. Physical management is difficult. Handling the baby causes tearing away of the skin, fluid loss, blood loss, and blister formation. Infection was a constant danger. Feeding was difficult because lesions were found in the mouth. Consultants from dermatology were unable to offer any curative treatment. They recommended only local skin care, and analgesics for pain. They advised against ventilatory support or resuscitation since this illness is so debilitating to the patient and care providers. Should efforts have been made to prolong the life of this baby? Was the intense pain of survival a greater evil to be avoided than the evil of death? Was the life of this newborn of sufficient value to it and/or others to justify the costs of its continuation?

Case C: A near-term baby was born to a woman who had no prenatal care. During labor, her uterus ruptured, resulting in the fetus being placed in her abdominal cavity. The newborn infant had no spontaneous respiration at delivery. It suffered from a prolonged lack of oxygen. Apgar scores were zero at one and five minutes, indicating an extremely poor probability of survival (Apgar scores are visual measures of appearance/color, pulse, grimace, activity/muscle tone, and respiration).[1] The baby was intubated and transferred to intensive care. Bleeding in the lungs and an absence of any electrical activity in the brain were observed. Appropriate interventions were begun. On day two, the

baby was breathing on its own, had some spontaneous movement, and a second EEG was no longer flat. The prognosis for
this infant, if it survived, was not clear. It was estimated that with
the prolonged hypoxia (insufficient supply of oxygen) the baby
would probably only have a vegetative existence. Perhaps it would
be unable, even, to suck to eat. The mother had six other children
at home. The family was indigent. The father was in jail. Should
the support of this baby be continued? Does human biological
existence with almost no reasonable prospect of being anything
else require continuation?

In each of these cases, answers to the questions depend, in
part, on the standing of newborn human life within the moral
community. The duties of beneficence owed to newborn human
life and the claims that such life can rightfully place upon others
are dependent, in large measure, upon their status as persons or
nonpersons. Efforts are underway among scholars to refine the
meaning of "person" in the belief that a clarification will shed
light on some of the difficult cases in bioethics, including cases
such as these. One purpose of these inquiries is to sort out what
we are obliged to do, what we are obliged not to do, and what
is purely elective, i.e., not subject to strict prescription or pro-
scription. Implicit to decisions regarding the care of any patient
is an understanding of personhood that, in effect, constitutes a
threshold below which rescue or life support is not obligatory and
above which there is a prima facie obligation to sustain life. (This
implied standard of personhood is roughly morally equivalent to
the notion of minimal independence discussed in Chapter 2.)

Understandings of personhood are variable in theory and
practice, reflecting particular moral commitments of individuals,
families, medical staffs, and communities. As biologist Robert S.
Morison observes regarding the seeming irreconcilability of diverse concepts of personhood, "If we are to have peace and mutual respect in contemporary society we may have to put the
veritable nature of personhood into the same category as the eu-
charist and allow each man and woman to decide where he or
she stands as a matter of conscience and religious liberty."[2] Insofar as Morison's comments are directed toward newborns and
those humans relevantly like newborns, the mutual respect he
advocates seems reasonable. A justification for this mutual respect will be developed during the course of the present discussion.

To determine what a "person" is requires insight from many disciplines since the character or nature of personhood appears so complex. We tend to approach the question of what is a person with a view of a fully developed, normal, human adult and, in order to determine the point at which one becomes a person, move backward to the initiating stage of those properties or property deemed sufficient for personhood.[3] At this initiating point, the entity is considered part of the moral community, subject to the same respect that is given to its more mature members. As might be imagined, much of the debate about personhood has taken place within the context of the struggle over abortion. Though abortion and the status of the fetus are not primary concerns here, there are important logical and conceptual links between the status of a fetus and the status of a newborn infant.

So-called pro-life advocates equate "human" with "person" so as to confer the inviolability of persons onto the fetus. Similarly, newborns would count as persons possessing a right to life and assertable claims for protection. However, an equation of this sort seems misleading both with regard to the fetus and with regard to the neonate. To say that both are human is to make a biological, descriptive statement. No one denies that a fetus or a newborn is human. It is not a dog or cat fetus or newborn. The species of the fetus or newborn is not the point of disagreement in these debates. Rather, at issue is the value, the importance that being human has in the moral community. As philosopher Charles Hartshorne observes, "To short-circuit consideration of the value question by equating 'human' with 'human in the full value sense' [person] is not a scientific procedure but a political maneuver or semantic trick that can only deceive those not trained to analyze arguments."[4]

As Hartshorne suggests, when used in a moral sense, personhood is a value-laden concept. What is and is not judged a person reflects basic value commitments that may differ remarkably. Some people wish to restrict the moral status of person to humans (referred to here as genetic theories of personhood). Others wish to focus on certain capacities or properties that some humans may not possess and some nonhumans may possess (referred to here as property-based theories of personhood). What is judged to be a person is important because the moral community is held to have duties to protect and sustain persons, and these differ from its duties to protect and sustain nonpersons.

Because the respective standards of these two theories reflect values that differ at such a basic level, it does not seem likely that either will be convinced by the arguments of the other.[5] Nevertheless, it is my observation that both understandings of personhood and moral duty are operative, at least intuitively, as decisions are made to attempt to prolong the life of an imperiled newborn or to accept its death. In order to illustrate how the concept of personhood is relevant to decisions in neonatology, like those required in the cases outlined, several efforts to define personhood need to be briefly summarized.

Genetic Theories of Personhood

As noted, some commentators equate "human" with "person." They hold what I call a genetic view of personhood. Genetic theorists argue that personhood does not depend on recognition by any particular society. They fear that this standard involves an arbitrary choice that is too subject to abuse. It is better, in their view, to consider all and only members of the human species as persons, and the decisive moment during development at which humans become persons is conception. It is at this moment that the genetic code of the new being is established. A human genetic code is held to establish a being as a person, " . . . a self-evolving being."[6] The inherent personhood that is created at conception becomes more and more manifest by a gradual process of biological, psychological and social development.[7] Personhood becomes more recognizable and perceivable as the potentiality embedded in the genetic code is realized over time. The value of human life, therefore, "does not depend upon a certain condition or perfection of that life." Accordingly, "all human lives are of equal value; all have the same right to life."[8]

An equation of human genetic endowment with the status of personhood can be challenged on several counts. No one disputes that the product of human conception is human. But the genetic view of personhood, when fully stated, moves beyond human biology to describe personhood. A person in the fullest sense of the term, as stated above, is "a self-evolving being." This suggests that persons are minimally, even according to this conservative view, capable of self-determination. Since human neonates are not capable of self-determination, according to this argument, they cannot be "fully" persons. Further, the worry about the arbitrariness of criteria other than species membership is flawed. This charge seemingly fails to recognize that limiting persons to members of the species homo sapiens is also arbitrary. (More will be said about this below.) In addition, the assertion that potentiality establishes personhood often has been challenged by the counter example that because one is a potential president of the United States does not require that he or she be treated like the commander-in-chief. Finally, an association of being human with a right to life is subject to the same charge of speciesism that can be directed against efforts to restrict personhood to humans.

Appeals to developmental biology do not establish moral status. To describe what is present and how it develops does not, in and of itself, automatically or by some logical necessity entail the status of personhood. Personhood and its appurtenant rights are ascribed or added to certain beings by culture. The designation of person is important primarily because it changes the way the possessor is treated by society.[9] Those who link humanhood with personhood are seeking to treat all instances of humanity, and only instances of humanity, with a degree of respect that may or may not be appropriate. An extreme interpretation of a genetic view of personhood would seem to require that the newborn human life described in cases B and C be prolonged to the extent possible. Case A might not require life-prolonging efforts because of the nature and severity of the defects. Further, extending life in cases B and C could be seen by some, even advocates of genetic views of personhood, as either pointless or cruel. It should be noted, however, that advocates of the genetic view are able to accept letting some patients die in particular circumstances. This allowance is achieved frequently by appeal to the principle of double effect, which attempts to preserve the life-prolonging presumption of moral rules by distinguishing evils that are intended from those that are not prevented or intended though foreseen.[10] Another justifying reason is to make a distinction between ordinary and extraordinary treatments. As will be explained, extraordinary interventions are not considered morally obligatory if they impose a grave burden on the recipient or do not offer a reasonable hope of benefit.

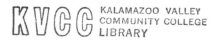

Property-Based Theories of Personhood

A second family of approach to the concept of personhood is non-genetic. Uncomfortable with the premises, reasoning, and conclusions of the genetic view, some commentators have given greater emphasis to certain attributes, properties, or qualities that establish an entity as subject to rights and duties, a being with its own ends, a person.[11] There is general agreement within this school that genetic humanity is irrelevant to a being's status as person. There are, however, differences regarding which property or properties are sufficient for personhood and secures a right to continued existence.

The preferred property or properties in one form or another relate to neurological capacities and functions. Joseph Fletcher, an ethicist who has written on medical ethics since the mid-1950s, considers neocortical function the essential trait or property of personhood. In his judgment, "without the synthesizing function of the cerebral cortex (without thought or mind), . . . [t]he person is nonexistent no matter how much the individual's brain stem and mid-brain may continue to provide feelings and regulate autonomic physical functions." Sapience, however minimal, "is necessary to *all* of the other traits which go into the fullness of humanness. . . . Without mentation the body is of no significant use."[12] Several philosophers also have addressed the question of what traits are sufficient for personhood. Mary Anne Warren thinks that three traits are central to the concept of personhood in a moral sense: consciousness and the capacity to feel pain; capacity to reason; and self-motivated activity. She finds that the first and second may be sufficient for personhood, but that all three are probably sufficient.[13] Peter Singer allows self-consciousness, rationality, and capacity to experience pain and pleasure to be relevant, but focuses on self-consciousness as the primary criterion.[14] Michael Tooley includes as persons only those substances or entities subject to nonmomentary interests or possessing the concept of a continuing self.[15] H. Tristram Engelhardt, Jr., favors self-consciousness, rationality, and self-determination.[16] It should be clear, according to the criteria adopted by these authors, that all newborn human infants fail the test for personhood. Therefore, according to this view, they do not have a right to life at all costs—financial, emotional, or medical. The life of nonpersons can have value, but not value of the sort that cannot be overridden by the needs and interests of others.

Normal human adults possess the relevant property or properties sufficient for personhood. They are persons in a moral sense. They are bearers of rights, including a right to life. Other creatures that possess the relevant properties similarly would qualify as persons. This leads Peter Singer[17] and Michael Tooley,[18] for example, to speculate that normal adult chimpanzees—and perhaps whales, dolphins, dogs, and cats—might possess the relevant properties for personhood. Killing them would be morally comparable to killing normal adult humans. Killing nonhumans or human life that does not possess the relevant person-making properties, according to this argument, would not be inherently wrong.

Even though newborn humans are not persons with full moral rights, property-based theorists are hesitant to give an unqualified endorsement to infanticide. Warren rejects infanticide on two counts. The first is that the destruction of an infant unwanted by its parents would deprive those who want an infant the pleasure of having it. Infants are like "natural resources" and "great works of art"; they can give pleasure. Their wanton destruction would be wrong. The second objection to infanticide turns on the presumptions that "most people" in this country value infants, favor their preservation, and are willing to be taxed to pay for their support. Given these conditions, Warren concludes that "it is *ceteris paribus,* wrong to destroy it."[19]

Singer would place strict conditions on what would count as permissible infanticide.[20] These conditions would apply more because of the possible effects on others than on the wrongness of the act itself. Infanticide and abortion are on a par for Singer when the parents do not want the infant or fetus to live. If the parents want their baby to live, its destruction would be viewed differently. Defective newborns unwanted by parents, and not likely to be adopted, could be killed under Singer's policy. Their species membership is irrelevant to their moral status. Their death would be viewed in the same way as that of any other sentient, but not rational or self-conscious, animal. When an infant's life is reasonably projected to be so miserable that it is judged not worth living, it is permissible to kill it. Such behavior is not morally equivalent, according to Singer, to killing a person.[21]

Tooley similarly rejects the claim that newborn humans are persons possessing a right to continued existence. He finds no behavioral evidence that newborns have higher mental capacities that would be essential for personhood according to his definition. All of these capacities emerge much later than the newborn period. Neurophysiological and bioelectrical evidence are seen to support these behavioral findings. At best, for Tooley, infants become quasi-persons at some time after birth, perhaps as early as three months of age. This age is selected on the basis of some evidence that a limited capacity for *thought*-episodes emerges around this time. The moral significance of this property is proportionate to the degree that it is present.[22]

Tooley concludes that "New-born humans are neither persons nor even quasi-persons, and their destruction is in no way intrinsically wrong. At about the age of three months, however, they probably acquire properties that are morally significant, and that make it to some extent intrinsically wrong to destroy them. As they develop further, their destruction becomes more and more seriously wrong, until eventually it is comparable in seriousness to the destruction of a normal adult human being."[23]

This general reluctance to give unqualified approval to infanticide seems to be explained by recognizing the social role that human infants have. Infants are not persons in a moral sense. They are not moral agents. They are not responsible or bearers of rights and duties. They are characterized by Engelhardt as persons in a social sense, "others must act on their behalf and bear responsibility for them. They are, as it were, entities defined by their place in social roles (for example, mother-child, family-child), rather than beings that define themselves as persons, that is, in and through themselves. Young children live as persons," he continues, "in and through the care of those who are responsible for them, and those responsible for them exercise the children's rights on their behalf. In this sense, children belong to families in ways most adults do not. They exist in and through their family and society."[24] Thus, newborns are valued not because they are persons but because they will grow to become persons, and because they have social roles *as if* they were persons.

Since infants are not persons in a strict sense, they do not have rights or duties except to the extent to which rights and duties are "exercised and 'held in trust' by others for a future time and for a person yet to develop."[25] Even so, Engelhardt does not propose that killing infants, normal or defective, is of no moral significance. Rules or policies that govern the treatment of newborns, who are not persons in a strict sense, "will need to be justified in terms of whether such practices will in general support the interest of persons in particular goods and values, including those of moral character." Another consideration for such a policy is the pain involved in the act of killing. These concerns lead Engelhardt to conclude that "human biological life [human nonpersons, e.g., fetuses and neonates] may be a moral object in a special sense, even when it is not a moral subject in the sense of a moral agent."[26] Killing an infant, all else being equal, is a serious act, but no more than killing an animal of a similar level of sentience. But for Engelhardt, all else is not equal because infants have a different "moral role within particular communities of persons." Imputing personhood to infants, that is personhood in a social sense, serves to establish general practices that "secure important goods and interests, including the development of kindly parental attitudes to children, concern and sympathy for the weak, and protections of persons in the strict sense when it is not clear that they are still alive."[27]

The general thrust of a nongenetic approach to personhood is more compelling, in my opinion, because it tends primarily to give greater priority to those properties of life that are basic to the possible experience of goods beyond that of vegetation. This is not to deny the good of biological human existence. Rather, it is to place it within the context of an infinite number of goods that necessarily are chosen among and rank-ordered. If human vegetative or biological life deserved absolute protection, as the gene-based theories of personhood claim, then it would appear that all other goods should be sacrificed in order to protect existing lives. It would seem also that the number of human lives should be increased without regard for their probable ultimate capacities in order to promote more good. One can imagine a world in which culture and nature were sacrificed to serve such an end. Such a world would tend not to promote the flourishing of those characteristics of life that secure one's place within the *moral* community (e.g., choosing freely among goods), as opposed to securing one's place in the *biological* community (e.g., maintaining vegetation). A property-based theory of personhood escapes the arrogance of speciesism and places humanity within an interdependent nature, broadening the scope of moral concern to include other life forms that may qualify for greater respect. It is no more arbitrary to identify one or more properties sufficient for membership in the moral community than to limit membership to humans alone, regardless of their development or capacities. Property-based theories can recognize the value potential without confusing and/or collapsing the rights of actual persons with the putative rights of potential persons.

A property-based theory of personhood seems to correspond with our moral reasoning regarding what we as moral agents owe one another. Decisions are commonly made that a patient's life and its capacities are no longer commensurate with the costs, broadly understood, of its extension. Duties of beneficence toward the patient are thereby defeated. A patient may reach this conclusion for himself or herself. Others may decide when a patient is unable to do so. Implicit in these determinations is a finding that, all things considered, the life that is lived no longer requires being sustained by the moral community in the form of efforts to impede the mortal process. The property or properties that once established the individual as a bearer of claims to beneficence may be irreversibly lost. Similar assessments could be made about entities that have not attained and will never attain the person-making property or properties, e.g., certain severely impaired human neonates. It does not violate the notion of the moral community[28] to conclude that some newborn human life does not possess a right to life, especially when person-making properties are beyond their capacity to develop or the costs of doing so are incommensurate with the probable good of prolonged life. It is possible that similar conclusions could be reached by proponents of genetic-based views of personhood. The duties of others toward a patient would not be determined by the patient's status as a person. Rather, it might be concluded that prolonged life is not in the best interest of the patient. One could determine, as well, that the treatments necessary to extend life would impose a grave burden on the patient. As such, they would not be morally required. It should be granted that this sort of reasoning can move one to a morally acceptable decision. It does not appear, however, to extend our scope of moral concern beyond humanity. Property-based theories offer an advantage over genetic-based theories in this regard. Property-based theories provide criteria to determine which nonhumans properly are objects of moral duty and which humans are not.

The specific properties identified by Fletcher, Warren, Singer, Tooley, and Engelhardt are subject to debate. Surely proponents of genetic-based theories of personhood would claim that the property-based standard for admission into the moral community is mistaken. They would not, I think, discredit the contribution that the proposed properties make to a robust existence. Their fears regarding an acceptance of that standard tend to be consequentialist in nature. That is, they fear what horrors the strong might impose on the weak or disvalued of our own kind if the protection afforded them is removed. What may begin as a reasonable exception to a strict prohibitive rule threatens to become less and less a reasonable exception, gradually engendering a disrespect for humanity on less than worthy grounds. This concern has merit. The injustices of the past should serve as a constant reminder that the weak are vulnerable to exploitation and abuse by the strong. However, as the past is recalled, it ought to be kept in mind that well-intentioned advocates of a genetic-based theory of personhood in reality can bring about, if successful, a tyranny of the dependent in which the production of able persons is consumed by the almost limitless needs of dependent beings. This more unusual form of tyranny is as equally subject to moral objection as a tyranny of the powerful over the impotent.

Another reproach against property-based theories is that they risk minimizing the cultivation of esteemed virtues. Compassion, sympathy, patience, courage, and loyalty, it could be argued, are in too short a supply as it is. The other-regardingness required by genetic-based theories guards against the loss of these virtues that express our care and concern for one another, even in times of weakness, vulnerability, and dependence. Proponents of property-based theories respond, however, that the free choice of persons to support nonpersons is not denied. The contribution of these virtues to moral life is endorsed. Not accepted, however, is the notion that a failure to protect nonpersons is in and of itself a moral wrong. Human biological life alone (fetus and neonate) is not a person, not a bearer of rights and duties. Its control is subject to moral agents most closely associated with it. The interest of the moral community in nonpersons is, ceteris paribus, minimal.

A final objection is religious. Based upon revelation, the claim is made that human life is a gift of God and therefore not subject to human judgments of its worth. Humans are endowed with value by God. As Creator, the Holy One owns life; it is only held in trust by humans. Good stewardship requires its perpetuation and enrichment. Innocent life ought not to be abandoned or ended as a result of human decision. Counterarguments turn on notions of responsibility under God. As beings with a free will, persons are responsible to one another and for creation. The reason with which God endowed humanity is to be exercised in ways that serve the good, not perpetuate or compound an evil. The value of human life, even all of creation, can be affirmed, but the obligation to make hard decisions in one's role as trustee or steward ought not to be forfeited. The divine imperative to love does not disclose what form such love should take in every historical instance. People who derive moral guidance from religious traditions probably simply decide, hoping to obtain God's favor, realizing that mistakes can be made, and believing that forgiveness is possible. The fact that life is innocent, apart from consideration of its person-making properties, does not, in and of itself, set it beyond human control. The lives of cattle, pigs, chickens, and lambs are innocent, but they are routinely ended without much, if any, moral anguish.

These brief comments, and those above, in response to genetic and property-based theories of personhood will not end the debate. Whereas genetic theorists might advocate life support for cases B (skin disease) and C (brain damage), property theorists would tend to view their nonsupport as permissible. Both camps would probably not require life support in case A (fetal tissue), even if such were possible. It should be clear that the property-based approach is considered by this author a better way to determine the moral status of human newborns. They properly can be considered persons in a social sense, even those with defects that foreclose the possibility of becoming persons in a strict sense, i.e., self-determining moral agents. The duty of parents and others to protect and sustain a newborn is proportionate to the probability of it attaining those capacities or properties sufficient for personhood. Clearly this view is at odds with the genetic theory that confers personhood on all and only instances of humanity. The duty to attempt rescue or to let die would be determined by genetic theorists on grounds other than the present or probable future status of the newborn, e.g., ordinary-extraordinary moral reasoning. The premises and methods that divide the two schools constitute a substantial hurdle between them that will not be easily cleared. Agreement may not be possible. The aim here was to indicate that the personhood of human neonates is a debated issue. As such, the rights of neonates, their status within the moral community, and the duties of persons toward them can be interpreted differently. Legitimate concerns are voiced by both sides. Each advances arguments in support of values that deserve consideration as decisions regarding the care of severely diseased or defective newborns are made. The freedom of both schools to adopt and act on their respective views ought not to be foreclosed. Until such time as an argument garners the assent of all parties, tolerance of reasonable individual determinations regarding the care of severely impaired newborns seems in order.

Implications of Conceptual Consistency

The concept of personhood has been debated mostly within the context of the problem of abortion where the focus has been on the status of the fetus. Nevertheless, participants in this conversation have been aware of the implications of their views for newborns. Genetic-based and property-based theorists see the fetus on a similar level of value and protection as the newborn. Abortion and killing neonates are seen morally by the two as related. Personhood is inherent to pre- and postnatal human life for the genetic-based school. Personhood is conferred by a decision of persons and the moral community for the property-based school. The most reasonable point to bestow personhood, in a strict sense, is at some uncertain point after birth when relevant properties are possessed.

The moral consequences of a conceptual link between fetus and neonate as espoused by right-to-life and quality-of-life advocates, rough equivalents of the genetic-based and property-based approaches, can be analyzed. The right-to-life view provides for equal protection of the fetus and neonate. The quality-of-life view protects adult self-determination over reproduction, pre- and postnatally, and the putative rights of newborn infants are subject to suspension in order to serve a higher social good. Commentators grant the consistency of both arguments. Some object, however, that ''an argument should not furnish principles for guidance in one situation (abortion) that could be used to destructive ends in another situation (euthanasia of neonates or terminally ill persons)."[29] But unless one reasons inconsistently, as long as the relevant features in two situations are materially similar, judgments, actions, and treatment with regard to them should be similar. This is a basic requirement of justice. It is not always easy, however, to know the criteria of similarity that warrants similar treatment of two entities, e.g., we kill rats in the street but protect them in the laboratory. If abortion can be justified for certain indications, those same indications should justify, at the parent's request, killing *newborn* nonpersons. This means that if a fetus is found to have spina bifida or Down syndrome, and these diagnoses warrant abortion, a *neonate* discovered to have spina bifida or Down syndrome at birth can justifiably be terminated. Yet it is this consistency that seems to trouble some people.

Those who are troubled by this conceptual and reasoning consistency view newborns differently from previable fetuses. Newborns, they argue, can exist without the support of the mother. Previable fetuses cannot exist without the consent of the woman whose rights and needs may conflict with the continued existence of the fetus. The capacity for separate existence, according to this view, constitutes a sufficient reason to sustain newborns who have independent moral claims to protection. The moral claims of previable fetuses, they admit, cannot be respected without disrespecting the needs and rights of the woman. In situations of conflict, the previable fetus yields to the woman but the viable fetus or newborn has equal standing. Thus, abortion of previable fetuses, with or without defect, can be accepted. Killing neonates, however, even those with defects that routinely warrant abortion, cannot be accepted because they are "fellow human beings," supportable apart from the mother.

This view places too much emphasis on viability in order to justify an inconsistency in reasoning. The newborn is still a dependent entity. Without the care and nurture of others it will die. The source of that care and nurture would appear irrelevant to a consideration of the force of the neonate's putative moral claim to beneficence. Nothing else, other than the neonate's physical place, seems to have changed. Its genetic endowment is the same. Its properties immediately before and after birth are the same. Why, then, does separate existence constitute a moral claim of greater magnitude? The answer, all things being equal, is that it does not. This sort of consistency in reasoning may cause some psychological discomfort, but such distress is not sufficient to create a relevant difference where none exists. One cannot have it both ways. One cannot advocate protecting viable fetal or newborn life without also advocating the protection of previable human life—not if one reasons consistently.

It is clear that this inconsistency also is represented in the law. American law considers birth to be the initial and death the terminal boundaries of personhood. Within this interval, the law states that each human being is entitled to all of the rights and statuses possessed by all other human beings. The law tends not to specify exceptions to this general rule. As Angela Holder, a professor of health law, remarks, "[I]ndividual variances normally cannot be accommodated because in many status situations it is more important that the law be certain and easily ascertainable than that it be correct."[30]

Legislatures and courts tend to define terms such as "person" with reference to a specific issue or for a particular purpose. Apart from the general presumption of the law concerning what and who counts as persons, however, it appears that the law is able to accommodate a standard of protection that takes account of relevant properties of personhood. For example, in the historic *Roe* v. *Wade* decision of the U.S. Supreme Court, fetuses were held not to be subject to state protection against the wishes of the woman during the first two trimesters of pregnancy. Similarly, in the case of Karen Quinlan, the Superior Court of New Jersey recognized that Ms. Quinlan's condition was such that her rights to beneficence were lost, but not her rights to forebearance, i.e., according to the law, her death could not be brought about by, for example, shooting her with a gun. These two highly publicized legal decisions suggest that courts can recognize that the life of some humans is of such low status that its prolongation is no longer required by the state. Decisions to this effect are perceived to constitute acceptable limits or exceptions to established legal principles. In a sense, the law is similar to moral reasoning grounded in genetic-based theories of personhood. Both are able to accommodate certain actions that otherwise would be proscribed apart from the extenuating circumstances of a particular case. Rather than being seen as misapplications of legal reasoning, they are viewed as expressions of judicial wisdom and mercy. If the property-based view of personhood were incorporated into the law, there would be no need to find exceptions to legal principles in order to authorize what is determined to be just and compassionate in particular cases. Some concept of personhood that is property-based seems implicit to these sorts of legal opinions. Furthermore, the use of property-based criteria does not seem to offend social values, particularly in cases similar to Karen Quinlan's.[31] If this perception is accurate, it seems that a more explicit judicial acknowledgment of property-based criteria is in order. Such an acknowledgment could serve two ends: it would help educate the public about the validity and utility of property-based theories of personhood, and it would help clarify our moral and legal obligations toward certain classes of patients.

In sum, the argument of property-based theories of personhood is that some forms of human existence are materially and morally different from others. The difference rests on certain properties possessed by some and not others. Only those entities possessing the relevant properties are considered full members of the moral community, bearers of rights and duties. The difference between persons and nonpersons permits different treatment. Genetic-based theories, on the other hand, deny that any property other than the biological one of human genetic endowment is necessary to establish membership in the moral community. Personhood is inherent, not imputed. Instances of genetic humanity are persons who have a right to continued existence.

It should be clear that one's understanding of what is morally required, forbidden, or permitted in response to the birth of a severely diseased or defective newborn can be influenced, at least in part, by the presuppositions, arguments, and conclusions of these theories of personhood. This is not to suggest that parents are intellectually aware of or seek to learn what scholars are saying about personhood when forced to decide for or against treatment. Nevertheless, some parents perceive the present life and potential future of their severely impaired newborn to be such as not to obligate them to authorize efforts to prolong its existence. Other parents may reach a different conclusion. In this sense, a concept of personhood, perhaps poorly articulated and only intuitively known, seems operative. An alternate approach to discerning what is morally required or allowed in these situations does not depend on a determination of the moral status of the newborn. It grants that the newborn human has standing in the moral community. The extent of a duty to sustain the life of a newborn depends on the perceived value of its life.

Value of Life

It is unusual for parents and care providers to appeal to concepts of personhood to justify a decision to attempt to rescue an imperiled newborn or accept death. It is much more common, in my experience, for some conception of the value of human life to inform their deliberations. This method of making treatment decisions presumes that the life of every infant has value. At issue beyond this presumption, however, is whether life is of sufficient value for the infant and/or others to justify the costs of its prolongation. Like the status approach (theories of personhood), there are two schools of thought regarding how the value of life is assessed (sanctity of life and quality of life) and one's moral duty in relation to that assessed value.

Common Concerns

The sanctity-of-life and quality-of-life approaches are sometimes expressed as moral principles that guide conduct. The sanctity-of-life principle assigns value to human life *regardless of present or future qualities or capacities*. This value generates a strong presumption that life ought to be sustained and protected unless there are overriding reasons not to do so. The quality-of-life principle assigns value to human life on the basis of certain *present or future qualities or capacities*. In short, the value of life is related to certain identified qualities. The duty to sustain life is related to the presence or absence of those qualities that confer value on a particular life sufficient to warrant its prolongation. Both principles or approaches to discerning one's moral duty to sustain an imperiled newborn have an interest in at least two types of information: medical "facts" (diagnosis and prognosis) and experience (pain and suffering).

Diagnosis and prognosis. The discovery that a newborn is not normal may require decisions regarding medical care beyond that usually provided to healthy newborns or to newborns with insignificant problems. Ascertaining that something is wrong may occur prior to birth (e.g., intrauterine growth retardation), at birth (e.g., congenital malformations), or soon after. Upon being informed that all is not well with their baby, parents want to know what exactly is wrong. In response, efforts are initiated to arrive at a diagnosis that in itself carries a presumptive therapeutic imperative.[32] An accurate diagnosis is critically important to the proper management of each case. The chance of some form of diagnostic error is always present. For example, an infant was reported by phone to have a Grade 3 bilateral intraventricular hemorrhage (bleeding in the ventricles of the brain on both sides one level below the worst diagnosis). The neonatologists began appropriate interventions to lessen the amount of brain damage and to prolong the baby's life. When the written report of the examination arrived in the nursery the diagnosis was Grade 4 bilateral intraventricular hemorrhage. A mistake had been made in the verbal report. Infants with the most severe diagnosis (bilateral Grade 4 IVH) often are not treated as aggressively since the neurological damage can have severe consequences for the survivor and its family or care providers. As in all fields of medicine, neonatologists and their consultants are responsible to provide competent care based upon the best available medical knowledge and evidence. They cannot be expected to do more nor permitted to do less.

An accurate diagnosis is necessary for a second reason. In addition to wanting to know what is wrong and what can be done, what this means for the probable future of the child weighs heavily in the decision to seek to prolong life, to allow death, or to hasten a mortal process (this last course is not presently permitted by law or sanctioned officially within the medical community). The diagnosis and prognosis, taken together, suggest something of the sort of life the newborn will have, if it survives, and the possible effect the baby's survival will have on others. Some diagnoses carry a fatal prognosis, e.g., anencephaly, Trisomy 13 and 18, renal agenesis—there are no effective interventions available. This sort of case can be excluded from consideration here since no decision will alter the ultimate outcome. Diagnoses for which there are effective therapies such as to reasonably anticipate a normal or not materially disvalued near-normal existence also can be put aside, e.g., hyaline membrane disease, most surgically correctable congenital malformations of the heart or bowel, infections, and mild hydrocephalus. These infants tend to have a high probability of future independence gained at an acceptable cost. It is extremely rare for anyone to advocate their nontreatment.

The cases in neonatology that are medically, legally, and morally perplexing are those in which the newborn's life might be salvable but (1) to a non- or minimally autonomous, non- or minimally relational, perhaps essentially biological level (e.g., prolonged asphyxia at birth); (2) is at a level of impairment that effectively renders life pleasureless (e.g., epidermolysis bullosa dystrophica); or (3) will be at a level of life purchased at an incommensurate cost (e.g., inborn metabolic defects). Less severe and more controversial instances of this sort of infant would be Down syndrome and spina bifida. The debate about life support for babies affected with these genetic defects (Down syndrome and spina bifida) tends to dominate the public and scholarly discussion about treatment decisions in neonatology. As important as these conversations are, they focus only on a relatively small number of cases within the total population of newborns about whom life or death decisions may be required. Premature, low birth weight, congenitally malformed, or diseased babies are representative of this larger number. Cases of this latter sort are the primary focus of this volume. Nevertheless, all cases of reproductive mishap challenge our moral intuition that life is an ultimate, inviolable value. They test our senses of justice, duty, and beneficence. In addition, they call for a judicious exercise of moral wisdom.

Diagnosis and prognosis constitute a factual basis, albeit subject to error and imprecise estimates of probability, that can place an infant in a class in which its death appears to some as the least among foreseeable evils subject to human choice. Everyone directly involved in these cases wrestles with the question of what course is required or justifiable in order to fairly attend to the interests of all concerned. In my experience, it is a rare exception rather than the rule for these troublesome cases to be approached by health care personnel or parents with a reckless disregard and insensitivity to the moral gravity of the decision that is required. The most frequent parental and medical response is a careful consideration of multiple concerns in a sincere effort to do what is considered appropriate. An effort is made to determine how the infant's present and future condition will bear on the value life has and will have for the child and those who are responsible for the child's care. In this sense, diagnosis and prognosis are utilized by both sanctity-of-life and quality-of-life proponents to discern what course morally ought to be followed.

Pain and suffering. A second factor that influences assessments of the value of life is the character of the experience of life for the child and others. In short, decision makers are concerned about the amount of pain and suffering that continued life portends for the infant and those who care for him or her. Pain and suffering are perceived as evils that ought to be avoided or lessened. When it is felt that an infant's pain and suffering are intense, unmanageable, or constitute an incommensurate cost for prolonged life, parents may view death as a preferable outcome (in an effort to protect their baby). Pain, suffering, and death each is disvalued, but their relative disvalue depends on the circumstances of a particular case. It is not unusual for parents to want their baby to live, but not if prolonged life entails pain and suffering perceived as intolerable, either as an effect of the disease's course or of the medical interventions necessary to extend life.

Pain and suffering, as evils, are relevant moral components of treatment decisions. They are within the purview of the moral principles of nonmaleficence and beneficence. The principle of nonmaleficence states that one ought not do a harm or evil to another.[33] The duties derived from the principle of nonmaleficence are negative in nature; that is, moral agents are restrained from acting in ways that harm or impose an evil. The principle of beneficence is concerned with the prevention, decrease, and/or removal of evil and harm. Because the duties of nonmaleficence are negative in nature, whereas the duties of beneficence are positive in nature, with respect to evil and harm, some ethicists rank the duties of nonmaleficence lexically higher than the corollary duties of beneficence. This means in practice that a duty not to inflict a harm or evil on someone is stronger than a duty to prevent or remove a harm or evil. A worrisome feature in neonatalogy is that efforts to save or prolong life may in fact engender more pain and suffering, a fate that might be considered more evil than death.

Parents and clinicians rarely distinguish pain and suffering. Pain is perceived to entail suffering and suffering is perceived to be caused by or related to pain. The two are seen as either corollary or synonymous phenomena and concepts. However, an equation of pain and suffering may be misleading. As philosopher Jerome Shaffer observes regarding pain, "[W]hen we try to understand pain—what it is, its causes and effects, its moral status, its place in our lives and in the world, its theological and metaphysical significance—we find pain to be not the simple and obvious phenomenon it seems at first but something extremely complex that remains resistant to analysis, understanding, and explanation."[34] The sort of inquiry indicated by Shaffer cannot be undertaken here. All that is necessary to note for present purposes is that pain, a sensation of a certain felt quality and intensity that evokes a negative attitude or response,[35] may be physical or mental. Newborn humans would seem capable of experiencing physical pain but probably not mental pain since mentation is beyond their capacities. Parents and care providers are capable of experiencing mental pains such as grief, loss, guilt, or sorrow, which also can produce physical pains, all associated with the predicament of a severely ill newborn. The relation between pain, either physical or mental, and suffering is complex. There can be suffering without pain (e.g., intense itching, a form of physical suffering; homesickness, a form of mental suffering) in which suffering is a "sense of distress or misery in some degree or other, . . . not caused by pain, either physical or mental."[36] Similarly, there can be pain without suffering (e.g., masochism). It seems, then, that suffering is related to the negative or disliked meaning or interpretation given to experience. Thus, family and care providers can suffer because of an incapacity to give positive meaning to experience.

These simplified distinctions suggest that a neonate's pain, but not suffering (since it is questionable that a neonate can suffer), is a morally relevant consideration in decision making. It is impossible, however, to know the intensity of pain that a newborn experiences. It may be inferred from a baby's behavior or projected onto an infant from the experience of more mature humans. The pain *and* suffering of parents, family, and concerned others are *also* morally relevant. The intensity of their pain and suffering can be known, presumably, since they are able to communicate. Like the baby's pain, the pain and suffering of relevant others are evils that ought not to be inflicted or compounded (according to the principle of nonmaleficence) and ought to be prevented, lessened, or removed to the extent possible (according to the principle of beneficence).[37] By recognizing that neonatal illness and defect can inflict evils on others, the scope of moral concern in neonatology must go beyond that of the newborn alone. And if property-based theories of personhood are correct, there may be sound reasons to have greater concern for the evils experienced by persons than for the pain experienced by a neonate. The neonate's pain would remain a relevant consideration, but it would be of no greater or less moral significance than the pain of other animals with similar capacities.[38]

Decisions to treat or not to treat tend not to be based on this sort of analysis of pain and suffering. Parents and clinicians often project themselves into the situation of the newborn, imagining the newborn's present pain and suffering, anticipating the pain and suffering that will accompany prolonged life, comparing these evils with the evil of death, and then deciding to fight against or accept death. The choice can be influenced by an individual's capacity to cope with pain and adversity that is projected onto the infant. It also can be influenced by an objective, to the extent objectivity is possible, evaluation of the net benefits expected to accrue from possible courses of action. It is not always possible to discern which influence is greater as treatment discussions proceed and decisions are made.

For example, two babies were in intensive care with the same diagnosis of hypoplastic left heart. In essence, the left side of the heart, which normally pumps oxygenated blood to the body, is missing or not sufficiently developed to function properly. Both babies were born at term to parents who had planned the pregnancy. One mother had six other children by a previous marriage, but this baby was the first child of her current marriage. The other mother was in her first marriage, and this was her first pregnancy. The only possible therapy for this defect is surgical, an operation called the Norwood procedure (named after its developer). Unfortunately, the consulting surgeons have never been successful with it even though they had tried several times.

The parents of both babies were told of the procedure, the surgeon's willingness to attempt it, their previous failures, and certainty of early death without a successful operation. The severity of this malformation is difficult for parents to appreciate during the first days of life. These babies look healthy and are reasonably vigorous. The parents of both babies understood the innovative nature of the proposed surgery. One family decided to attempt the surgery and the other family refused. The surgical patient died in recovery. The second baby died within two days in intensive care. The parents who rejected surgery explained their refusal this way: The baby would surely die without surgery and probably would die with surgery. The mother said, "If I were Johnny and likely to die regardless of what is done, I'd rather not go through the pain and suffering of surgery first." Ironically, the mother of the other baby explained her choice for surgery this way: "It's his only hope. And if it were me I'd try anything, regardless of the pain and suffering involved, to live." Clearly, pain and suffering were important, if not decisive, considerations for both sets of parents.

Physicians, too, are concerned about pain and suffering. The medical maxim "do no harm" expresses succinctly medicine's aversion to impose unnecessary pain and suffering upon patients. The pain and suffering associated with an intervention is weighed against the expected benefits for the patient. In neonatology, these assessments are more properly directed toward the pain to the infant and the pain and suffering of others, including the members of the neonatal team. They, too, may experience pain and suffering, during the course of care for a newborn, in a manner similar to that of parents and family members. In short, pain and suffering, are evils that are to be prevented, removed, or lessened. Critical cases in neonatology almost inescapably involve pain and suffering. Yet determining the level of pain and suffering that each party experiences can be a problem. The predicament can become even more perplexing when the pain and suffering of the respective parties must be rank-ordered and chosen among.

The perceived level of pain and/or suffering that a newborn experiences or generates for relevant persons can influence judgments of the value of the child's life and the moral duty to attempt its prolongation. The relative weight given to the experience of the infant and its impact on others tends to vary among families and care providers. This is to say that in some cases the focus with regard to pain and "suffering" is exclusively on the infant. If the value of life is judged a net benefit for the infant, life-prolonging interventions are undertaken. If life is believed not to constitute a net benefit for the infant, death is seen as a grace. When the scope of concern is broadened to include the experience of others, as well as the imperiled infant, similar judgments to attempt to save or to accept death can be reached. Here the infant's value of life is weighed in relation to the gain or loss of value to others that the infant's life portends. Decisions to attempt to rescue or to allow death will reflect a judgment that continued existence of the infant constitutes a net benefit or loss to those parties materially affected. The infant's life is not valued in isolation. Rather, it is one value in relation to and comparable with the value of the lives of persons who will be materially affected by the imperiled newborn.

Perceptions of pain and suffering, together with an understanding of relevant descriptive (diagnosis) and predictive (prognosis) data, clearly are relevant to value of life judgments. These forms of data and assessments, as indicated above, tend to be considered relevant for decisions whether one follows a sanctity-of-life or quality-of-life approach. For a sanctity-of-life ethic, this information is critical in the determination of whether or not the strong presumption to protect and sustain human life can justifiably be overridden. For a quality-of-life ethic, this information is critical to determining whether or not those capacities believed to make life worth living are present or probably will be attained. The scope of concern may be limited to the infant's life or extended to include materially affected others, principally parents and siblings. How a sanctity-of-life and quality-of-life approach incorporates these and other matters into decisions to treat or not will be analyzed more fully in the next two sections.

Sanctity of Life

As noted above, the sanctity-of-life view values human life independent of its capacities, holding that human dignity, worth, and sanctity are from God (in its religious form) or is naturally inherent (in its secular form). The religious form of this view is dominant. Roots for the sanctity-of-life principle can be found in the Judeo-Christian tradition. Judaism and Christianity affirm that the value of human life comes from God. It is not based upon or derived from some quality, capacity, trait, or property of life. The value of life is not subject to human decision. Life is understood as a gift from God, held in trust by the one who lives it. Others are responsible under God to protect, enrich, and prolong life. Human dominion, according to this view, is legitimately exercised when it aims at the preservation, not the destruction or surrender, of life. These beliefs provide a foundation for the principle of the sanctity of life. All principles, including the sanctity of life, provide general guidance. Thus at times their meaning for specific cases can be elusive. In addition, there is a tendency, especially with sanctity of life, for principles to be reduced to slogans used in emotional support of different causes, e.g., the so-called right-to-life movement.

In its extreme form, sanctity of life is expressed as where there is human life, regardless of its condition or the individual's wishes, it would be wrong to let life end. Proponents of this view are fearful that any principle less restrictive than an extreme interpretation would weaken compassion and charity for the disadvantaged. They worry that if exceptions are allowed to a strict rule to prolong life, the floodgates will be opened to all sorts of abuses. Human decisions to accept death or end life may be described as playing God. In their view, only God determines when life properly ends.[39] A final worry focuses on the role of medicine. Extreme sanctity-of-life advocates argue that the emphasis of medicine should be on prevention and cure, not surrender to death or the destruction of life.

A less rigid interpretation of this principle stops short of a near absolute valuation of earthly existence. While agreeing with the general themes and thrusts of the principle, more moderate proponents of a sanctity-of-life ethic hold that there is a prima facie, not absolute, obligation to protect and preserve human life. Designating the obligation as prima facie implies that there can be legitimate exceptions to the general rule. They grant that God is the author of life, but attach the claim that persons are co-creators with God, responsible to make considered judgments regarding it. Biblical notions of dominion and stewardship are interpreted to direct human activity toward bringing order out of chaos, relieving pain and suffering, and minimizing evil. Moderates point to a contradiction of extremists when God's absolute dominion is affirmed and killing in self-defense or during a just war are defended. Moderates respond to the charge of playing God by observing that the phrase is selectively and polemically used only against those who are willing to accept death. Like some parents, moderates ask how one can know that efforts to prolong life clearly in a terminal stage is not contrary to God's will, a form of usurping God's position, a form of playing God?

While holding to the main theme of the principle of the sanctity of life, moderates approach difficult treatment decisions in a manner similar to that of quality-of-life proponents. They are able to do so by appeal to a distinction between ordinary and extraordinary means of preserving life. From a moral point of view, "*or-*

dinary means of preserving life are all medicines, treatments, and operations, which offer a reasonable hope of benefit for the patient and which can be obtained and used without excessive expense, pain, or other inconvenience."[40] Antibiotics, for example, administered to a newborn with an infection and who is otherwise healthy would be considered ordinary means of treatment. Extraordinary means of treatment would be those interventions "which cannot be obtained or used without excessive expense, pain, or other inconvenience, or which, if used, would not offer a reasonable hope of benefit."[41] Antibiotic therapy for an acute infection in an infant with multiple organ failure would be extraordinary. The benefit to the infant would be negligible since death would soon come as a result of organ failures totally unrelated to the acute infection.

Characterizing interventions as ordinary or extraordinary grows out of a moral tradition, principally Roman Catholic, that was concerned to determine the extent of one's duty to submit to or to provide medical treatment in order to prolong life. Stated simply, ordinary treatments were considered obligatory and extraordinary treatments might be considered elective. While it was generally agreed that moral agents ought to avoid doing what is intrinsically evil (e.g., murder or suicide), there was disagreement regarding the limits of the duty to do good (e.g., prolong life). Moralists understood that one's duty to do good was circumscribed by reasonable and proportionate limits. They sought to define these limits with regard to prolonging life by answering the question, "How much does God demand that I do in order to preserve this life which belongs to God and of which I am only a steward?"[42] As the above formulations of ordinary and extraordinary indicate, the answer was framed in terms of expense, pain, and other inconveniences.

One was not obliged to impose a great financial hardship on oneself or family in order to live longer. Such a burden was seen to reflect more than a "reasonable" care of one's health and, therefore, not required by God. Similarly, procedures involving great pain could be foregone. Major disruptions of one's life (e.g., moving to another climate) also were seen to go beyond God's demand to preserve one's health or life. Accordingly, actions judged to produce excessive expense, pain, or hardship to self or others were considered extraordinary and not morally required. When this was not the case, the means to preserve life were considered ordinary and morally required. In like manner, interventions that offered no reasonable hope of benefit were termed extraordinary. Interventions that offered a reasonable hope of benefit were called ordinary. The former were not morally required; the latter were. A treatment is ordinary, according to this line of thought, if it can be obtained and used without significant inconvenience and if it offers a reasonable hope of proportionate benefit. When either of these conditions is lacking, the means is extraordinary.[43]

Newborn infants are not capable of making this sort of judgment regarding treatment. The claim in this volume is that parents are responsible to speak on behalf of the child. As the definition of extraordinary acknowledges, the burdens that can properly be considered in making these judgments include those imposed on others. The expense, pain, and inconvenience of treatment on relatives, for example, are also worthy of consideration. Assessments of the burden of treatment are not limited to its impact on the infant patient. Parents or others acting on an infant's behalf could decide that the interventions believed necessary to prolong an imperiled infant's life would impose a grave burden on the child or its family. In these instances, life-prolonging treatments would be considered extraordinary, not morally obligatory. This decision could be made while fully holding to the concept of the sanctity of life. The value of human life is affirmed. Yet some people reason that there can be circumstances in which the net value of life to an infant and/or to its family is disproportionate to the burden necessary to prolong life. As such, efforts to extend life are judged extraordinary and not morally required.

Quality of Life

The quality-of-life approach, like the sanctity-of-life view, affirms that human life is a value, but its worth is limited. Human life is a basic, conditional good of instrumental value. It is necessary to the experience of other goods, harms, and evils. Judgments of what makes life worth living can change over time and in response to changed circumstances, facts, and values. Advocates of a quality-of-life approach search for and weigh or order the features, qualities, properties, or capacities of human life that make it of worth for the one who lives it. This process does not necessarily entail sacrificing the lives of some for the lives of others on the basis of arbitrary, irrelevant, indefensible, or ill-considered reasons. As in the sanctity-of-life approach, human life is valued; however, unlike it, proponents of quality-of-life standards are more likely to embrace reasons other than self-defense or just war to justify taking or surrendering life. For example, one could argue that the pain of a neonate with a devastating skin disease (i.e., epidermolysis bullosa dystrophica, case B) outweighs the value of continued existence to the infant or to its family. Life itself can be seen to constitute a harm necessary to an evil. Given these conditions, proponents of quality-of-life standards of decision making could favor allowing the baby to die or terminating its life as morally licit responses.

No one disputes that quality-of-life judgments are value-laden. Similarly, everyone is aware of the uncertainty that necessarily attends this type of decision for someone unable to express his or her own wishes. Nevertheles, decisions are made, either to prolong a life of questionable value or to accept a grave loss for the peace of death. Judgments regarding quality of life, in addition to being value-laden and case specific, are also context dependent. This is to say that the environment in which a newborn will be placed can influence its projected quality of life. The quality of life in certain institutions or homes which lack the commitment and capacity to help that life attain its potential value would be different from the quality of life in other institutions or homes in which the commitment and resources are readily available. Issues of social justice are relevant here but will be set aside. Parents, neonatologists, and other surrogates must make decisions in light of the way things are, not what they ought to be. Quality-of-life considerations, in my experience, influence treatment decisions in all cases except those in which the relevant parties follow an extreme version of a sanctity-of-life ethic.

If environmental factors are relevant to quality-of-life judgments for newborns, then it is reasonable to consider the impact a severely defective or impaired newborn will have on its family, particularly if home care is chosen. The reordering of family life, plans, and goals necessitated by the presence of a newborn, who probably will remain in a newbornlike, dependent state regardless of how long he or she lives, can constitute a serious disruption to the normal course of life. Some parents worry about the effect this child will have on their marriage and the opportunity costs to present and/or future brothers and sisters. Parents either provide the level of additional care, including the probable costs to the family, that the natural lottery has placed upon them or they seek some form of relief through social programs, institutionalization, surrender of custody, or death of the newborn. Whichever course is taken there are costs to pay along the way. Marriage, family life, and the welfare of other children are relevant, and at times competing, goods worthy of consideration as the present medical care and probable future of a severely defective newborn is being decided. Taking account of the interests and needs of others, or even giving them priority over the limited but absorbing prospects of the neonate, does not constitute an abuse of the strong over the weak. A decision in favor of one over another is not discriminatory unless there are no relevant differences between them. In my opinion, an incapacity to attain a minimal level of independence or to become a person are relevant differences that warrant decisions favoring marriage and siblings at the expense of the neonate. This sort of hard choice is not sought by parents, yet it may become one of several options occasioned by the birth of a severely impaired or defective baby. Surely parents and siblings are and ought to be free to surrender voluntarily their present and future well-being in order to care for the new member of the family. But it is by no means clear what level of sacrifice is morally required.[44]

One could argue that there are no guarantees in life, that pregnancy by nature is risky, and that unless prospective parents are willing and able to accept the outcome, good or bad, they should remain childless. This argument has merit in that it underscores the serious responsibilities of parenthood. Parenting entails general commitments to protect and nurture the new being. At issue, however, is the notion that these general commitments are unlimited and irrevocable. Few other choices in life, short of successful suicide, bear these qualities. Spousal love fails, friends part, debts are renounced, and contracts are disavowed. Good faith pledges to perform specific acts may be determined impossible or too onerous to fulfill. Socially acceptable mechanisms have been developed to sanction actions that enable people to "cut their losses," e.g., divorce, institutionalization, and bankruptcy. It seems reasonable to think that analogous formal procedures could be devised that would sanction a limitation or revocation of the customary parental duties to protect and nurture defective newborns who meet carefully defined criteria. Court refusals to order certain medical procedures that would prolong life are indications of the formal possibilities. The acquiescence with which these decisions regularly are met in hospitals indicates that an informal possibility may be a reality already. Lastly, one could respond that parents do not seriously consult with or obtain the consent of present children when planning to enlarge the family. If present children do not agree to the risk, should they be *required* to pay the cost? Membership in any community, by birth or choice, implies some sharing of the benefits and burdens of that community. Adversity has as much potential to weld relationships and commitments as it does to sever them. But it seems intuitively unfair or unjust to sacrifice the opportunity of a healthy child in order to sustain the existence of a severely defective or impaired brother or sister. The concerns of parents for their marriage and other children are legitimate. Each entails commitments and duties that deserve consideration. The putative duties of parents to a newborn can be weighed against those duties already in place. When the costs to sustain the newborn are found incommensurate with the net goods to be gained, decisions against the newborn in favor of others seem morally permissible.

However quality-of-life decisions are approached and regardless of the concerns taken into account, in my experience, there is a tendency toward what might be called a neurological bias. Parents, neonatologists, and others seem to focus on the brain as the key organic indicator of whether the newborn's life ought to be prolonged to the extent possible or whether the newborn's death ought to be received as a grace. An emphasis on the brain is understandable. It is the key organ in humans related to the capacities sufficient to establish one as a person. In addition, the brain integrates bodily/organic functions, through its sensory functions the world is experienced, and from its intellectual and emotional capacities we reveal who we are. The vital significance of brain function to one's standing in the moral community has been legally and medically recognized and affirmed by whole brain definitions of death. Additionally, a focus on neurological status and related capacities or potential seems to reflect the value that culture places on intellectual achievement. When a baby has a "bad head" there seems to be a greater willingness to see death as a reasonable alternative to vegetative life. When a baby has a "good head" there seems to be greater willingness to see life as better than death.

The inclinations or dispositions implicit to a neurological bias can reflect personal, medical, and social judgments regarding a life worth living. But there is a danger in normativizing neurological capacities and potential for decisions to save or let die. That danger is to forget, ignore, or minimize the potential of other impaired vital organs to diminish the quality of life to the one who lives it and its value to others. Cardiac, renal, hepatic, and bowel abnormalities, in addition to being potentially lethal, can be so severely restrictive or debilitating that continued existence may not be considered an advantage. At times it is necessary to be reminded of the integrated nature of the human body without unnecessarily diminishing the strategic role of the brain. All relevant data deserve consideration in making treatment decisions for newborns. Reductionism of any sort risks oversimplifying medical and moral dilemmas of profound significance.

Conclusion

It is possible for parents to clarify their duties toward an imperiled newborn by means other than an appeal to the moral status of the infant as a person or nonperson. This alternate method, characterized here as a value-of-life approach, discerns duty on the basis of a perceived and projected value associated with the life of a newborn human. Two principles can guide this assessment of duty (sanctity of life and quality of life), but, as the discussion shows, it is possible that similar decisions can be made. This is to say that the reasoning associated with each principle can lead to similar judgments of whether life prolonging interventions are morally required. One decides, according to the sanctity-of-life principle, on the basis of the net value of life to the infant and/ or others. The basis for the decision according to the quality-of-life principle is the presence or probable attainment of certain qualities that are held to make life worth living. Both the sanctity-of-life and quality-of-life principles articulate concerns that are important to the moral life (respect for human life and appreciation of certain capacities that enrich human existence, respectively). For this reason and because both forms of the value-of-life approach are serious, valid efforts to reason morally about cases where clear guidance is lacking, reasonable judgments made in accord with either principle, in my opinion, deserve respect. Clearly my preference is the quality of life approach because it roughly corresponds to the main features of property-based theories of personhood. Nevertheless, the sanctity-of-life tradition, like genetic-based views of personhood, is able to provide competent moral guidance for situations of reproductive tragedy. This is especially true, in my opinion, when the sanctity-of-life principle is interpreted in a moderate, rather than extreme, manner. Genuine respect for the presuppositions, arguments, and conclusions of both value-of-life principles would appear to foster an atmosphere in newborn medicine of moral humility and tolerance. The task of determining what is morally indicated in these contexts can be difficult. Moral insight and guidance ought to be welcomed, regardless of its source, as contributions toward licit decisions. The prospect for morally valid decisions can be enhanced if certain procedures are followed and if certain possible influences are understood. It is to these factors that this discussion of the process of making decisions now turns.

Components of Decisions

It should be clear that the arguments contained in this volume are primarily concered with supporting the responsibility of parents to make reasonable treatment decisions, and generating greater mutual respect for morally valid decisions without specifying for every conceivable case what constitutes a valid judgment. In short, the aim is to establish parental authority in a moral pluralism. This concern, however, does not negate an interest in procedures that would appear to enhance the quality of the process and of decisions. But a reliance on procedure alone would not seem to generate the understanding and mutual respect necessary to life in a moral pluralism. The following section contains suggestions regarding how the task of deciding might proceed. In addition, the possible role that certain "nonfactual" factors may have will be examined. These comments and suggestions are offered in an effort to enhance the prospect that a valid decision is made and to indicate the role that noncognitive influences may have. Perhaps this discussion will contribute to the greater understanding and mutual respect that goes beyond that which can be achieved by a reliance on procedure alone.

Disclosure and Comprehension

In order for reasoned and informed treatment decisions to be made, it is necessary that the medical facts, as they are known at any given time, be communicated to parents, or other responsible parties, in a comprehensible manner. This means that the neonatologist's description of what is wrong, what interventions are possible, and what are the probable outcomes must be in terms that genuinely convey an accurate account of the situation. These verbal exchanges ought not to be seen as meaningless rituals that placate anxious and/or bothersome parents. Rather, they should be seen as precious opportunities to establish bonds of trust so crucial to a harmonious relationship between parent and care provider. Physicians and parents can come to know each other during these periods of disclosure, question, and answer. The family situation, moral commitments, religious beliefs, and values of parents can be discerned by physicians and taken into account as the care of the newborn proceeds. Similarly, parents can develop a confidence in or distrust for the medical team as they are perceived as either understanding or insensitive, competent or incompetent. By being informed and by understanding what has been communicated, parents are empowered, at least in principle, to make decisions based on a realistic understanding of their baby's condition and probable future.

At times, parents ask questions to which definite answers are not known. For example, how retarded will my baby be? How severe will the handicap be? How many operations will be required? How long will my baby live? Despite the qualifications that must attend almost any predictive reply, parents may be given answers that sound as if they are based on substantial experience. This is unfortunately not always the case. The ability to save the lives of some newborns who otherwise would have died without modern medical care is so recent that long-term outcomes simply are not known. At best, these predictions are educated guesses that will be revised over time as these babies are followed. Another possible limitation often not disclosed is the nature and quality of the evidence upon which certain statements are based. For example, the fact that current medical wisdom is based on a published study of only a few successful cases may not be mentioned. Also, other reports of less satisfying outcomes may go unmentioned altogether. Finally, there is the ever-present personal, perhaps single, experience of the treating physician: ''I had a case three years ago with the same problems that your baby has and now that kid is as healthy and normal as any other three-year-old.''

As these comments suggest, a physician's personal bias or professional ego can unintentionally color the facts so as to lead parents to a favored decision. The injection of personal and professional values, expressed or hidden, into conversations with parents about the present condition and future of their baby may be unavoidable. But if parents are to be enabled to make decisions consistent with *their* considered moral commitments, the full picture should be presented, and personal bias ought not to be passed off as medical truth. The accurate disclosure of information in a comprehensible manner constitutes a heavy and legitimate burden on those who possess it. The uncertainty that may be a part of answers to questions of anxious parents ought not to be glossed over. When such is the case, parents deserve to be told that there is not enough experience with a particular diagnosis to make a definitive answer possible. Alternatively, they could be told the nature of the experience that has been reported. At other times a particular diagnosis may lead to a range of outcomes so varied that clinicians properly should respond with statements of probabilities.

The uncertainty that attends these situations can be distressing to everyone involved, parents and care providers alike. The presence of uncertainty, however, does not relieve the responsible parties from making hard decisions. Neither does uncertainty warrant withholding relevant information, as it is known, from parents. Further, there is the chance that the best available medical evidence may prove wrong for a particular case. The legitimate exercise of parental responsibility requires that clinicians fully reveal all diagnostic, therapeutic, and prognostic data that can be reasonably considered important *to parents* as they make decisions regarding the care of their newborn. They have a need and right to be informed about what is known about the condition and probable future of their newborn.

In addition to the full disclosure of relevant information, competent decision making is enhanced by a functional comprehension of medical data. Clinicians may think at times that parents cannot bear unpleasant news, will not or cannot understand what is revealed, or cannot appreciate the significance of the disclosures. These are legitimate concerns. Care and concern for parents are valid considerations for the timing and manner with which information is communicated. Compassion for parents dictates that their grief not be compounded by a heartless, brutal pronouncement. Language can both comfort and destroy. It can communicate or obscure reality. Informing parents about likely outcomes for their baby may involve a version of show and tell. Visits to custodial institutions or with parents of children similarly situated may help parents to appreciate the implications for their child and family of what is being told to them. These discussions aim to equip and empower parents to make informed decisions regarding their child. Extensive amounts of a clinician's time may be necessary to help parents come to terms with the reality of their situation. The parents' preconceived ideas or fantasies about the consequences of a diagnosis may be far worse than is warranted. Similarly, uninformed or naive understandings may be far too optimistic. Asking parents to indicate what they understand about their baby's condition can help clinicians determine the degree to which parental decisions are medically informed.

Assessment

Value terms can creep into conversations. Good, bad, dreadful, dismal, and poor are value terms. Their use reflects the speaker's evaluation of a situation that may not correspond with the hearer's evaluation. The criteria and referents for these evaluations are rarely disclosed or explained. They tend to be shorthand expressions for a much fuller clinical picture. Specificity is a virtue in conversations with parents because of the prospect for misunderstanding. Rather than saying that a baby probably will have mild handicaps, why not identify those probable deficits, e.g., will not walk, talk, see, hear, control bladder and/or bowel? The parents can then assess the impact of probable deficits or handicaps according to their situation and values. A child with a projected maximum I.Q. of 40 may be less disadvantaged in a family where the average I.Q. is 90 than in a family where the average I.Q. is 140. The costs to maintain a severely impaired child may have profound negative implications for the opportunities of siblings in a low-income family, whereas the opportunity costs may be negligible in a high-income family. The meaning of an impairment, defect, or handicap is relative to individual contexts and desired ends. Parents and families, more so than intensive care personnel, will live with the consequences of decisions to treat or, perhaps, to let die. As such, parental judgments of good, bad, tolerable, or intolerable warrant thoughtful consideration by neonatologists as management decisions are made.

The ability or desire of parents to cope with a defective newborn ought not to be prejudged. I remember a vigorous debate with a neonatologist who refused to give parents the option to take a neonate home to die. The justification for the refusal was that the intensive care staff was accustomed to death. Besides, "why place an additional burden on the parents?" My argument was not with the apparent benevolent intent of the neonatologist. Rather, it was with a steadfast refusal to even inform the parents that taking the baby home before its death was possible. Some parents value very highly taking their terminal baby home as an indication of its place in their lives and their love for the infant. They might also value being able to perform such basic parental tasks as diapering, feeding, and bathing that were denied to them while the baby was in the hospital. Signs that the baby's death is near could be explained. The infant then could be returned to the hospital to die or it could die at home. The point is that parents almost without exception should be free to make the choice.

Classifying Treatments

In addition to the medical facts, their comprehension, and their evaluation, another typical feature of the process of decision making is a tendency to use terms such as ordinary, extraordinary, and heroic to describe interventions.[45] These terms convey the speaker's sense of the moral requiredness of a specific intervention or course of interventions. As noted earlier, ordinary care means interventions judged obligatory, required, or mandatory from a moral point of view. Extraordinary or heroic care means interventions judged morally optional or elective.

Often specific interventions are mistakenly considered ordinary or extraordinary in and of themselves. Rather than classifying an intervention in terms of the net balance of benefits and burdens expected with its use in a particular case, there is a tendency to categorize specific interventions regardless of the circumstances of a particular case. For example, respirators may be judged extraordinary and antibiotics ordinary interventions. But in terms of net benefits, ventilation would be ordinary care for a baby with hyaline membrane disease (lungs not fully developed due to prematurity) and extraordinary care for a baby with anencephaly (absence of brain). Antibiotics would be ordinary care for acute infections in newborns without other life-threatening problems or severely handicapping defects. They would be extraordinary care for a newborn with no brain, a fatal condition.

Ordinary, extraordinary, and heroic designations of care, when used properly as case- and treatment-specific terms, indicate an estimate of an intervention's relative contribution to certain attainable treatment goals and, accordingly, their morally required or optional status. When these terms are misapplied or used without a common understanding of their meaning the decision-making process becomes complicated, confused, and usually physician-dictated. Rather than expressing a considered judgment about the efficacy and relative value of a specific intervention, these terms when misused express an intuition, preference, or desire that may not reflect historic ethical understandings and applications. When utilized accurately, the process of decision making can be simplified and more focused. Achieveable ends can be identified, possible interventions can be examined, and appropriate judgments regarding their moral requiredness can be made.

Psychological Influences

In addition to these procedural and linguistic elements that can confound the process of decision making, psychological factors can have a complicating role. Everyone involved brings to these hard cases their own professional, moral, and nonmoral values that influence, if not determine, personal views of what end and course is morally indicated. The judgments reflect one's vision of the good and the life worth living. However derived, these commitments constitute the core of one's moral being. They warrant respect by others in the moral community who expect an equal regard for their considered moral judgments. Unfortunately, an atmosphere of mutual respect for competing moral visions and the defensible judgments of right and wrong derived from them does not always exist. Overt or latent conflict can result. An interested party may universalize his or her moral judgments. Not only is a particular opinion considered right for the one who holds it, but others are expected to hold it, and only it, as well. A pediatric colleague exemplifies this tendency to universalize one's values and moral judgments. She holds that good parents are those that are willing, even eager, to prolong the life of a child regardless of the handicaps the child may have and regardless of the burden imposed on the family. Good parents, in this colleague's judgment, never surrender a desire for their child to live. Giving up, accepting or desiring a child's death, even for reasons of mercy, are viewed as selfish actions.

A tendency to universalize one's values and/or normative judgments also can run in the opposite direction. Parents, especially those in professional occupations, may expect clinicians to share the values that shape a decision to treat or not to treat an impaired infant. When values and choices are not shared, parents in professional roles may be intolerant of the clinician's judgment. They are, at times, unable to understand why professionals like themselves would not or could not appreciate and comply with their decision.

The potential dangers of this sort of universalization of values and norms are magnified in situations in which the conflicting parties do not exercise equal power. The stronger party is positioned in these circumstances to impose upon others a personal moral judgment that may be no more or less justifiable than that of another party. This can be the case in health care relationships, particularly in pediatrics. A physician's personal values and moral judgments can be medicalized, presented as if they express standard medical practice or wisdom. Recommendations based on nonmedical value, moral, or religious commitments may be given the authority of medicine. As a result, parents who have been schooled to accept medical wisdom regarding their best interest, may accept these recommendations without questioning their source or possible alternate courses of action. Challenging a neonatologist's advice risks being belittled as a bad parent or being taken before a judge for alleged neglect of a sick newborn. Fortunately, these sorts of confrontations are rare in my experience. Reasoned disagreements that surface are subject to compromise. At other times, the baby will either die or get better, rendering an unpleasant confrontation unnecessary or changing the nature of the decision that is required. Nevertheless, the potential disruptive role of universalizing and normativizing personal values should be recognized and guarded against.

The final psychological factors to be commented upon are identification and projection. Care providers, especially neonatologists, nurses, and social workers, seem prone to identify with the needs, desires, and preferences of parents. They project themselves into the situation of the parent, imagining themselves to be in the parents' situation. This sort of projection and identification can engender sensitive expressions of concern, sympathy, compassion, and support. It can also lead to a shifting of patients. The parents become the object of primary concern, not the impaired neonate. Rather than holding in balance the interests of all concerned, the scales of decision making are tilted so as to either give priority to expressed parental desires or to effect an end considered by the medical team as best for the parents. Two cases illustrate how an identification with parents can influence behavior.

A thirty–two-year-old woman had tried unsuccessfully to become pregnant during the entire period of her ten-year marriage. Finally she became pregnant but the course of her pregnancy was complicated. She started labor during the twenty-second week of the pregnancy and delivered a 17½-ounce (500-gram) baby. At the parents' insistence, every effort was made to save the life of the newborn even though the medical opinion was unanimous that it was not viable. The mother and father were charming people. They were extremely kind to the medical team and appreciative of their efforts to save the baby's life. The parents were almost constantly in the hospital during the three days of the baby's life. Despite multiple confirming signs that this newborn was not viable (e.g., no urine output, and the death of skin tissue), every effort was made to prolong its existence. The sole reason for doing so was to satisfy the wants and needs of this likable couple. The clinical staff empathized with the parents desire for this infant to survive. Out of concern for the parents and imagining what they would want if in the parent's situation, they attempted to save the baby's life even though they did not think that this was possible.

The second instance of identification was reported in Chapter 3. The parents had one adopted child and were adopting a second baby only days old. Unfortunately, the baby developed herpes encephalitis and other neurological, cardiac, and respiratory complications. This perceived kind and generous couple was felt by the neonatal team to be trapped in a situation they did not deserve. The care that would be required if the baby survived was considered an unfair burden to impose upon these people, who were perceived as self-sacrificing parents. As a result, the medical care of the baby tended to be less aggressive in a seemingly unconscious effort to protect the parents from an avoidable injustice.

This is not the place to debate the merits of the neonatal team's motives or actions in either instance. The cases are intended to illustrate how psychological factors can influence treatment decisions. Yet they are not intended to suggest that only the medical staff is subject to psychological influences. Parents can project motives for behavior onto clinicians. They may believe that vigorous efforts to save the life of a severely impaired baby are designed more to enhance a physician's reputation than to advance the best interest of the newborn. As might be expected, in situations like this, the decision-making process can become extremely contentious, taking on an appearance of combat rather than cooperation.

Religious Beliefs

The decisions that are required of parents and others during a child's severe illness can be agonizing to all. Faced with a hard choice that might be inconsistent with basic parental inclinations to protect and nurture, parents frequently seek the care and counsel of their pastor. Theological doctrines and concepts can help shape the medical care decision that is required.[46] A pastor, rabbi, or other religious authority can confer with the family, provide a theological interpretation of experience, give meaning to meaninglessness, explain the moral wisdom of their religious tradition, and mobilize the support of fellow congregants. The burden of decision making can be lessened or increased as a result: lessened if decisions are compatible with religious teaching and/or medical opinion, increased if decisions are contrary to religious teaching and/or medical opinion.

Beliefs, commitments, and values of ultimate significance to the parents can be challenged in these critical situations. The involvement of religious authorities in consultative and comforting roles should be no surprise. As options are explored and decisions are made, parents can receive from or through their pastor, rabbi, or religious authority divine sanction for the course taken. Such approval can lessen the prospect for feelings of guilt or shame, whether the choice was to accept death or struggle against it. Prayer by the crib and religious symbols in or on the crib provide links to the caring religious community of which the family is a part and to the concern their god holds for them even in their distress. Healing, intercessory prayer, and other religious rituals and expressions by members of religious communities provide symbolic participation in the infant's and family's care. The importance and power of religious beliefs, commitments, and values to shape parental responses ought not be underestimated or ridiculed. Some of the more poignant expressions of parental love and concern for a severely ill newborn that I have seen have been clothed in religious symbolism. I offer two examples.

It was the fourth pregnancy for the couple. The earlier attempts to become parents had resulted in miscarriages. A baby girl was born five weeks premature, weighing 66½ ounces (1,900 grams), and diagnosed with hyaline membrane disease, which is not unusual for preemies. The prognosis was good for recovery. However, after admission to intensive care the baby's condition deteriorated unpredictably and rapidly. Her kidneys failed. On day four of life, the baby had a cardiac arrest, was resuscitated, placed on a ventilator with 100 percent oxygen and high pressures. Cardiotonic drugs (Dopamine and Isuprel) were given to increase blood pressure, urine and cardiac output, and pulmonary blood flow. On day six, a pneumothorax (air in chest) led to a second cardiac arrest. The baby was again resuscitated. Chest tubes were inserted to relieve the pneumothorax. Within twenty-four hours additional pneumothorases led to a third arrest. Resuscitation and more chest tubes followed. On the seventh day of life, the baby was found by ultrasound examination to have a bilateral grade 4 intraventricular hemorrhage (severe bleeding in the brain). Ventilation continued with an oxygen level of 100 per-

cent. By day twelve of life, the infant developed hydrocephalus
(fluid in the brain), which was not immediately treated because
of the other complications. On day fifteen, unsuccessful efforts
were made to shrink the ventricles of the brain with medication.
Further, the baby was considered too unstable for repeated spinal
taps to relieve the fluid buildup in the head. By day twenty, the
infant was blue and unconscious. All support systems were in
place.

The family had been told three times that death was imminent. At each point the baby survived. The parents, especially
the father, interpreted these events as signs that God wanted the
baby to live. Further, he became extremely concerned that the
medical staff would give up on the infant and allow her to die.
The father assumed a protective role, sensing that the medical
and nursing staffs were prepared to accept the baby's death. The
parents did not believe the negative reports of the infant's condition. Each movement and response to procedures were interpreted by the parents as encouraging signs that the baby would
live. The neonatologists were instructed to do everything possible
to save their daughter's life. At the same time, they purchased
burial clothes for the neonate and discussed with the staff whether
contact with a funeral director should be made then or upon the
baby's death.

The medical staff had a difficult time working with these parents. The mother spoke of her suffering and felt that the baby
was also suffering. Yet both parents desperately wanted the baby
to live. They asked for experimental procedures if the neonatologists considered them potentially helpful. The parents were
members of a conservative Christian denomination. They maintained that God intended for this baby to live. Religious symbols
adorned the crib. Their pastor visited daily and prayed with them
by the bed. A Bible was placed at the baby's side. A note to the
doctors and nurses was hung in a prominent place on the crib.
It read: "Thank you for taking such good care of my baby. Promise me that you WILL NOT give up on her even if things seem
impossible or at the end. Remember that God can ' . . . do im-
measurably more than all we ask or imagine . . . ' [Eph. 3:20].
I'm praying for you and Mary. Squeeze her little hand hourly for
me and tell her mommie loves her and she will be alright! God
bless you!'' Around 2:30 one morning, when the baby's death
was anticipated for the third time, the father stood by the crib

and wept while the baby struggled to live. Quietly he removed the note, walked the full length of the unit, and into the hall. He returned immediately and replaced the note. His comment was, "I thought that I had better put this back. We've not given up. God has not given up. And we don't want you to give up." Despite all efforts the baby died on the twenty-first day.

The second case involved a Down syndrome newborn with a congenital heart disease. During a spinal tap the baby's brain herniated. The baby suffered strokes, and swelling of brain tissue. All of this took place on Monday. The baby's condition grew worse each day. By Friday the parents requested that the baby not be resuscitated in the event of an arrest. They had decided that God did not want this baby to live. The neonatologists, according to the parents, were "in God's way" with all of the medicines and procedures. They preferred for the baby to live but if the newborn died they would be comforted knowing that it would be "born again in the Kingdom of God, healthy, whole, and happy. And the family would be together in heaven when they all died." The parents viewed the baby's death as a temporary separation and a blessing for the baby. The parents, who had one other child, were perceived by the neonatal team as loving and caring, and enjoyed support from family and church friends. When the baby died the parents were at peace. They believed God's will was done.

This is not the place to debate the validity of the religious convictions represented in these cases. However, it is clear that in these instances religious beliefs and values determined the parents' behavior. As suggested by these case reports, the involvement of religious authorities tends to be welcomed by health care personnel. It can have a calming effect for people in turmoil. At other times medical care can be complicated by an infusion of religious beliefs, especially those beliefs opposed to generally accepted medical practices and therapeutic values, e.g., Jehovah's Witness refusal of blood transfusion.

The procedural, psychological, and religious factors briefly reviewed here demonstrate that deciding the care of defective newborns is not a purely scientific, rational, or objective endeavor. The process of decision making is subject to influences beyond factual understandings. The terms employed to describe and evaluate an infant's condition, efficacy of possible interventions, and anticipated future have potential to bias decisions for or against treatment. In addition, the web of relationships formed around the medical care of an imperiled neonate can generate psychological phenomena that can influence the character of the decisional task and the conclusions reached. It is, therefore, mistaken to think that the present debate about the treatment of severely defective newborns can be settled by reaching a consensus about moral rules, the moral status of newborns, or the value of human life. Clarity and consensus about these matters would contribute to a better understanding of the issues and values represented in these troublesome situations. But solutions that are insensitive and nonresponsive to the personal and interpersonal features of these cases are incomplete and probably unsatisfying to the participants and to others concerned about these issues.

CHAPTER

6

To Kill or Let Die

THE PRECEDING CHAPTER SHOWED how complex, complicated, and potentially contentious the process of making decisions regarding the medical care of severely compromised newborns can be. The particular problems of the neonate coupled with the moral and nonmoral concerns of those individuals responsible for its care constitute a matrix of concerns that may not be easily or comfortably negotiated. I have argued that parents are the deciders of choice, duty, and right. They are responsible for making a reasonable judgment on the basis of a careful review of all relevant considerations, and, as they choose, in consultation with selected experts and authorities. They may elect to pursue treatment in an effort to preserve life and protect its potential or to accept death as the lesser evil.

When a parental decision intends action believed futile or abusive of a neonate, the neonatal team could reasonably resist cooperation. The communication between physicians and parents, however, usually is such that this sort of refusal is not necessary. Alternatively, when parents reasonably authorize efforts believed capable of sustaining life, the neonatal team has a prima facie obligation to implement their wishes to the extent medically possible. A parental decision and medical response of this sort tends not to evoke substantial moral pause because it corresponds with, on the one hand, a presumption for life and treatment, and, on the other, a view of the proper exercise of parental and medical

duties toward a newborn. These parental decisions and medical
performances intended to prolong life will not be evaluated here.
Rather, this chapter examines those parental decisions that foresee and/or intend the death of a severely diseased or defective
newborn, particularly one reasonably believed never able to attain a minimal level of independence or personhood. I have argued that these infants especially are subject to the authority of
parents. Destined by the natural, and perhaps to a lesser extent
the social, lottery to nonpersonal existence, disvalued life, or a
prolonged death if life-sustaining procedures are begun, these infants present a profound dilemma to parents, neonatal teams, and
the broader moral community: Should they be allowed to die or
may death be effected in a merciful manner? In order to offer an
informed answer, we shall consider the practice of infanticide and
the alleged moral distinction between killing and allowing to die.

Infanticide

The practice of infanticide tends to be viewed with horror by people in so-called civilized societies. The killing of infants for whatever reason is seen today by many as a relic of our dark, distant
moral pasts from which we have evolved and ought never to return. Yet the dark past of infanticide is not so distant. As anthropologist Laila Williamson reminds us, "Infanticide has been
practiced on every continent and by people on every level of cultural complexity, from hunters and gatherers to high civilizations,
including our own ancestors. Rather than being an exception,
then, it has been the rule."[1] To observe that infanticide has a long
history and that it has been widely practiced, however, does not
help us to reach a moral judgment regarding it in the past or proposals to accept some form of it in the present. In order to understand better why infanticide has been practiced and to discern
how the past informs the present, if at all, we shall consider three
categories of explanatory factors. Two caveats, however, should
be mentioned before undertaking this analysis.

The first qualification is definitional. Scholars have not always
distinguished killing a newborn from an older infant. For example, Williamson defines infanticide as "the deliberate killing of a
child in its infancy, up to two years of age,"[2] an age limit much

above the focus of this volume. It is difficult, as a result, to discern if parents and cultures that practiced infanticide viewed the killing of infants during the first month of life differently from those killed later. Further, efforts to determine the incidence of neonaticide versus killing older infants are burdened by the definitional imprecision in the relevant literature. Finally, all intentional deaths of infants tend to be classified as instances of infanticide. Killing by omission is not distinguished from killing by commission, a distinction that will be discussed in the next section. Thus it is difficult to be certain exactly what the literature means by the term "infanticide." This, in turn, complicates the process of making a moral judgment about infanticide in the past. Further, the light that historical precedent may shed on the current debate about killing defective newborns is obscured.

The second qualification stems from another form of imprecision. The historiographical research on infanticide is such that it is impossible to be quantitatively precise as to the degree to which infanticide was practiced in any given period and place. Often the most one can say is that, on balance, the evidence that has been discovered indicates that infanticide was more or less widely practiced at one time or place than at another. But it is difficult to know with certainty how frequent or widespread infanticide occurred. The fact, however, that we are reduced to this kind of comparative approach to the subject does not invalidate the analysis. For here we are primarily concerned with the factors that have served to explain the practice of infanticide, rather than with quantitative comparisons.

It should also be mentioned that certain of the explanatory factors that have been cited in the literature on infanticide can be classified as *reasons* for the practice only in the retrospective sense of reason. For example, it has been said that infanticide has from time to time served as one mechanism for keeping population size roughly in line with available economic resources. Thus, regulation of population size can be used as a reason that explains retrospectively certain factors about the prevalence and acceptance of infanticide among certain peoples at certain times. But in many cases it seems unrealistic to impute such factors to the relevant peoples as conscious, motivating *reasons* for what they did, either as individuals or as groups. The certifying data simply do not exist. We simply cannot know with certainty in every instance why a particular person or people practiced infanticide. At best, perhaps, scholars have had to settle for informed hypotheses to explain the practice.

With these qualifications in mind, three kinds of explanatory factors can be discerned from the literature. The first category explains why people were willing to practice infanticide. The second and third categories explain why the practice was tolerated, accepted, and rationalized. More specifically, the first category includes factors that, in the absence of impeding influences (such as the prospect of personal guilt, social ostracism, and legal punishment), render the deaths of certain infants a more attractive option than their continued existence. The second category includes psychological factors that mitigate the impeding influence of personal guilt. The third category includes legal and social conveniences that mitigate the impeding influence of such factors as social ostracism and legal prosecution or punishment. The lines between these three categories are not always sharply drawn. As will be seen, there has been considerable interplay between factors of one type with factors of another type. Nevertheless, the proposed divisions point to differences between various types of explanatory factors that have, in the literature, tended to be lumped together. These differences become especially important when the historical study undertaken here is seen as a backdrop to contemporary issues of neonatal life or death.

Why Infanticide

The factors that disposed people to infanticide can be grouped into three categories: economic, physical, and sociocultural. Economic factors are given a prominent place in the literature. The attempt to restrict the number of people alive, either normal or impaired, at a given place and time to a total roughly compatible with available resources for sustenance has been posed as an explanatory factor for infanticide at both the societal and the familial level. At the societal level, the importance of economic factors in the explanation of infanticide has been described for primitive societies by anthropologist Williamson.[3] Moreover, she has used economic factors also to explain the preference for selective female infanticide among such societies by indicating that female infants, since they are potential childbearers themselves, were seen to pose a greater threat to the sufficiency of a community's resources than male infants. Further, in some primitive societies, such as the Eskimo, the provision of food depended on the availability of a large number of male hunters. Thus, rearing female infants was seen as a threat to future food supplies, a perceived threat sufficient to warrant their selective destruction.[4] Similar appeals to insufficient economic resources as partially explaining at the societal level the practice of infanticide have been offered for the Middle Ages[5] and for early modern Europe.[6]

Availability of economic resources and related factors also have been used to explain individual acts of infanticide at the familial level. Williamson, for example, points out that among primitives, infanticide performed on a newborn, normal or defective, was often seen as an act of caring or regard for the older children in the family, since it forestalled an unacceptable drain on resources that were needed to sustain the others.[7] This explanation undercuts the popular view that, when it has been practiced, infanticide was an act of utter disregard for the rights and well-being of children. In this perspective, infanticide is more properly understood as the result of deliberations under conditions of scarcity in which concern and regard for the well-being of older children are allowed to outweigh the interests of the new arrival. Similarly, among migratory peoples, since a woman was better able to care for only one infant at a time, infanticide in cases of multiple births can be seen as an attempt to keep the number of infants requiring care in line with the amount of care available from an individual mother.[8] In Europe, during the long period from the Middle Ages through the nineteenth century, intrafamilial economic factors were responsible for many infanticides, particularly in cases of illegitimate births. A major reason for this was that the full economic burden of caring for babies born out of wedlock fell on the mothers,[9] even though during most of this period it was all an unmarried women could do to take care of herself. Thus, the added economic burden of child-rearing was a strong factor that inclined many unwed mothers to eliminate their children.

The second category of factors that disposed people to commit infanticide are physical—more specifically, physical factors that were related to abnormalities of the newborn. At various times, abnormality of an infant has been viewed as a sufficient reason to kill it. The destruction of abnormal infants in many primitive societies has been described by Williamson.[10] The practice of eliminating defectives became institutionalized in classical Greece and Rome. It was almost universally practiced, not prohibited by law, recommended in the political writings of philosophers such as Plato,[11] Aristotle,[12] Seneca,[13] and Plutarch,[14] and it was advised in ancient medical texts such as Soranus of Ephesus's text on gynecology.[15]

During the Middle Ages, a whole mythology developed concerning defective infants. Deformed and retarded children were termed "changelings," nonhuman creatures who were substituted by demons for a real infant soon after birth. The prescriptions within the myths for recovering the normal, healthy infant often resulted in the cruel killing of the defective infant. These methods were aimed at coercing the "powers" to return the stolen infant.[16] As ridiculous as this understanding sounds to modern ears, it apparently was commonly accepted during the Middle Ages. Other theories about defectives included the view that an abnormal infant resulted from the mother having seen or thought about "improper" things during pregnancy, and the view that "monsters" resulted from unnatural sexual liaisons between the mother and an animal.[17] In both instances, infanticide was recommended as a means of expiation for the mother's guilt.

The third category of factors that disposed people to commit infanticide are sociocultural. Among primitive peoples, the practice of infanticide in connection with sacrificial rites seems to have been fairly common.[18] In cultures with a ranked caste social order, such as India, infanticide has been practiced as a means of protecting the purity of genealogical lines.[19] And in cultures in which dowries were paid at the marriage of females, the selective infanticide of females was often employed to save the family this expense.[20] Finally, illegitimate offspring, in some societies, prompted a social ostracism of the mother, particularly when the offspring were of mixed blood. Thus, illegitimacy and products of interracial sexual unions have been objects of infanticide, particularly among, but not limited to, primitive peoples.[21]

Until very recent times, then, infanticide has been deemed a more attractive—and more effective—method of achieving a desired end than its principal competitors: contraception and abortion. In addition, it was much safer for the physical well-being of the mother than were the various techniques of abortion. Moreover, unlike abortion, infanticide allowed for the selective elimination of offspring for a specific reason, e.g., gender.[22]

Mitigation of Guilt

We turn now to those factors that explain the lessening or absence of guilt or blame that might be expected to attend the practice of infanticide. Two distinctions seem to be drawn that, in effect, mitigate the psychological burden of guilt. One is the view that, in some way or ways, the killing or letting die of infants is not as wrong as the killing or letting die of older humans. This view has taken at least three distinct forms. First, among many primitive peoples, it was held that a child was not fully human until the time of formal acceptance as a member of society.[23] Often this acceptance was signaled by the public performance of a ritual at the culturally acceptable age, which ranged from a few days to several years.[24] Second, a distinction between infants and older humans has been supported by superstitions and quasi-religious beliefs. Among certain primitive peoples the belief prevailed that, when a child was killed because of economic pressures, for example, its soul was not destroyed but rather lingered, awaiting rebirth at another, and hopefully more propitious, time and place.[25] Thus, the killing of an infant was less serious than the killing of older humans since the infant's soul would have another chance at life. Within Christianity, Augustine's view, which became the Catholic teaching for centuries, is radically unlike this primitive belief. For Augustine, the chief evil in infanticide was not that it deprived a child of life, but rather that it irremediably deprived a soul of the possibility of redemption through baptism, and thus barred its salvation.[26] Nevertheless, even in medieval Europe, infants—especially illegitimate or defective infants—were accorded less than full *legal* status. For example, in medieval England the penalty for the accidental killing of an infant was about half as severe as that for the accidental killing of an adult.[27] Additionally, myths such as the ones described above not only permitted but even exhorted the parents of defective infants to destroy them. The parents would, according to the myths, be blameless for their action. The third and final support for a distinction between infants and others emerged during the nineteenth century. A view was articulated by utilitarian-minded thinkers that "the killing of babies who are not old enough to experience fear is different from the murder of adults."[28] Presumably, different means less seriously wrong,[29] and infanticide was seen in this light because the act was evaluated in terms of the

net good or evil consequences it effected. The evil consequences
that attend the killing of an infant (both direct, physical consequences to the infant *and* consequences for the relevant family
and society) were considered less serious than those that attended the killing of an adult. Whence it follows, for a utilitarian
at any rate, that the former killing was less seriously wrong than
the latter.

The second distinction that assuaged the consciences of those
who practiced infanticide rested on a difference between acts and
omissions. There were practices whereby parents could "put out"
unwanted children under the presumption that their new guardian would either kill them or let them die of neglect. Death under
the oversight of a wet nurse, even though foreseen or perhaps
intended, incurred little or no blame as compared to that which
would have resulted if death came by the hand of a parent. In
Renaissance Italy, for example, a financially stretched mother
could hand her child over to the *balia* (wet nurse), with every assurance that it would soon be dead, and yet be subject to less
intense feelings of guilt than if she had directly killed the infant
herself.[30] The presumption that the infant would soon be dead
might, after all, be false; the wet nurse *might*, contrary to expectation, provide good care for the infant and rear it. In either case,
the mother could feel at least in part as if the baby's fate was out
of her hands.

Legal and Social Conveniences

The final factors that facilitated the practice of infanticide are those
legal and social conveniences that mitigated the impeding influences of social ostracism and legal retribution. A variety of legal
factors historically have rendered infanticide less risky than other
forms of homicide. Possibly the most extreme legal factor of this
kind was the Roman right of *patriae potestas*, which accorded the
Roman father absolute authority over the members of his household. Until the fourth century A.D., this right included the power
of life and death over a young child. Prior to that time, legal pro-
hibitions of infanticide ordered by the father were thought to be
an unjust infringement of the state into the sphere of paternal
discretion and liberty. Even after the prohibition, in A.D. 374, of
all acts of infanticide (with a death penalty for violation), it was

only *direct* killings of infants that were proscribed. Exposure and abandonment were not prohibited, presumably on the grounds that, in any such indirect killing, the remote possibility existed that the exposed child could be found, taken in, and reared by someone else.[31] The distinction between direct and indirect killing of infants also had a role in classical Greece, exposure being the method most often condoned and practiced.[32] However, " 'adoption' may not always have been better than death in ancient times, because the adopter often mutilated the children and made them into beggars who excited laughter and pity by their grotesque shape."[33]

Under the influence of Christianity, infanticide was outlawed throughout the later Roman Empire, though enforcement of the laws was difficult. For instance, while the direct and willful killing of an infant was a capital crime, accidental killings were punishable by much lesser penalties, such as a few years on bread, water, and vegetables, and abstinence from intercourse for one year. But it was difficult to prove that an infant had been willfully destroyed, particularly during the Middle Ages when it was customary for small children to sleep in their parents' bed. Accidental overlaying was a fairly common occurrence, resulting in the death of the infant. It was doubtlessly fairly easy for an infanticidal parent to intentionally suffocate a child and claim that it was an accident.[34] Later, in mid-Victorian England, a similar enforcement problem arose: "To prove 'neonaticide,' the intentional killing of a child at its birth or soon thereafter, one had first to demonstrate that the baby was born alive. But verification of live-birth, especially where the only witness to the act was the mother suspected of murder, constituted one of the most vexing problems in forensic medicine."[35] The fact that willful infanticide was a crime not easily proven, its commission was rendered less risky than other homicides. It should be added, as well, that the preponderance of successful prosecutions for willful infanticide involved unwed mothers,[36] which suggests that enforcement may not have been uniform. Fathers were rarely charged with the crime, and married mothers often were acquitted either on the plea of accident or by appeal to temporary insanity. Thus, because of an uneven enforcement of the existing laws, infanticide was less risky for fathers and married mothers than it otherwise might have been.

Social sanctions seem not to have been any greater a deterrent to infanticide than the law. In Renaissance and modern Europe,

a host of social institutions arose that facilitated the elimination
of unwanted children by their parents. The *balie*, professional wet
nurses, of Renaissance Italy already have been mentioned.
Though these women often performed the valuable service of
breast-feeding and caring for the children of upper-class families,
they also frequently, and increasingly as time went on, became
agents of death for infanticidal parents. Moreover, while infanticide by the hand of the mother was punishable by death, if committed by the *balia* the punishment was much less severe. And
since most *balie* lived in rural areas, far from public scrutiny, the
difficulty of obtaining a conviction was more pronounced. Thus,
as Maria Piers, professor of child development, has written, "For
all practical purposes, the wet nurse was assigned the role of the
killer-with-impunity."[37] Even as late as the mid-nineteenth century in England, historian William Langer reports that "Women
employed in the factories and fields had no choice but to leave
their babies in the care of professional nurses, sometimes called
'killer nurses,' who made short shrift of their charges by generous
doses of opiates."[38]

The great surge in the population of Europe from the mid-
eighteenth to the mid-nineteenth centuries resulted in hunger,
unemployment, and illness for ever-increasing numbers.[39] It also
resulted in a growing number of abandoned infants (many of
whom were illegitimate), in response to which philanthropic individuals and/or governments increased the number of foundling
hospitals, the largest in Paris, London, and St. Petersburg. The
demand placed on these hospitals by poor women seeking to be
rid of their children were so great that they quickly became over-
crowded. Insufficient space, medical care, and wet nurses resulted in high mortality rates.[40] Langer has written, "There was
no mystery about these matters. Mothers who left their babies in
the box [at the hospital] knew that they were consigning them to
death as surely as if they had dropped them in the river."[41]

This overview of the practice of infanticide may or may not
be disturbing. It could be read as a record of willful individual
and social moral failure. The explanatory reasons could be judged
either singly or in toto as inadequate explanations and insufficient
justifications for a practice that offends not only one's moral sense
but also the basic moral laws by which people of goodwill are to
live. The perceived relative disregard for infant life could be
viewed as despicable evidence of a human propensity to place

self above others, even those others who are defenseless and for whose existence one is responsible.

The inabilities or failures of conscience, custom, and law to impede a practice that seems inconsistent with our basic moral impulses could be seen as a cause for moral despair. In addition, one might regard the foregoing account as an indication that our savage, unenlightened past is more recent than we care to admit. In fact, some may worry that the sentiments that led to and allowed the practice of infanticide to exist for so long have not been sufficiently extinguished to ensure that it will never be taken up again with tacit moral and legal acceptance. The very fact of this history and the explanations discovered in its support could be perceived as an indication of the entrenched moral corruptions of humanity and society. As such, people of moral conviction might find this account so portentious as to warrant an erection of legal, social, and moral barriers sufficient never to permit, in the language of Vatican II, this "unspeakable crime"[42] to be committed with impunity ever again, regardless of the reason, explanation, or justification offered in its defense. One could conclude, accordingly, that this overview provides absolutely no moral guidance regarding treatment decisions for defective newborns except that any act which indirectly or directly intends or achieves an infant's death constitutes a moral wrong, similar to an immoral precedent, which should be judged as such and effectively prohibited.

On the other hand, the historical record could be read with less moral chagrin and outrage. One could view the circumstances, causes, and explanations with sympathy. Though retrospectively the practice, in general, might be viewed as regrettable, it could be understood, given the societal and cultural forces at work during any particular time and place. Individuals and cultures that engaged in, tolerated, or advocated infanticide could be regarded as not necessarily moral rogues but as people in crisis attempting more or less conscientiously to find their way. Though their moral lights might have been different from those prevailing today, their efforts to resolve a dilemma could be judged by the social realities and moral standards of their day and not ours. And unless self-righteousness moves one to a too-quick and absolute judgment, perhaps one could project oneself into the contexts and worldviews described herein and ask if one's action and judgment would have been markedly different from theirs.

The practice of infanticide could be understood as an indication of moral, social, and legal limitations that perhaps have been overcome with the passage of time. The perceived failings of our ancestors might be interpreted as evidence of their finitude, moral and otherwise, that is characteristic of all people in all times. One might not regard the record with pride and a desire that it be repeated in every detail, but one might accept it with humility and study it to discern what moral sensibilities exist within it to inform us as we confront moral dilemmas of similar substance and importance. Accordingly, one might derive some guidance from the record with regard to the moral quandaries that may be forced upon parents and the moral community by the birth of a severely impaired infant.

Historical precedents, either of practice or explanation, do not necessarily validate a contemporary activity or judgment. The medical atrocities under the rule of Adolf Hitler do not warrant analogous misdeeds for a subsequent regime.[43] Similarly, one cannot justify proposals to let die or to kill severely diseased or defective newborns by a simple appeal to the precedents described above. This does not mean, however, that this review is irrelevant. Rather than leading to normative conclusions regarding the medical care of neonates, it leads to certain understandings of the sort of people we are and the sort of communities we constitute.

The most significant lesson to be learned from this analysis is that people throughout history have determined that death for certain infants, on balance and for putatively sufficient reasons, was preferable to their continued life. It is clear from this history that newborn infants, in general, throughout time, have not possessed a moral trump card that mandates a preference for their interests over the interests of all others. The history shows that adults in situations of need have been disposed and able to balance the interests of a newborn against the interests of others, however those respective interests were defined. Contemporary efforts to confer upon newborn life, and fetal life as well, an absolute value appear to be abberrations within the human and moral record. The circumstances and nuances of the dilemma regarding the life or death of a defective newborn may be different today, but the contextual character of the process of deciding and the necessity to decide seem comparable. This is to say that decisions regarding the destiny of a severely ill newborn are not made in a vacuum. The contingencies and exigencies of social life, as well as the diverse and dynamic moral senses of the relevant agents, influence judgments that are made.

A second lesson that can be gleaned is that societies not only have been reluctant to intrude, they have been able to accommodate infanticide when done for socially acceptable reasons. Social peace seems not to have been destroyed even though segments of the moral community officially disapproved of the practice. Social conveniences developed to serve two ends: first, to facilitate the practice, and second, to protect certain values, such as the presumption of parental protection of children. Thus, for example, the use of surrogate agents of death served both ends. Additionally, the circumstances within which mothers or parents perceived a need to remove an infant from their care probably were seen as chaotic, disproportionately burdensome, or meaningless. Myths and pseudoscientific explanations seemed to bring some order to the perceived chaos, and mitigated whatever personal guilt that might have attended a decision to rid oneself of the burden. Though the myths and other efforts to explain the natural and social lotteries would not be accepted today, analogous explanations (e.g., God's will, medical explanations of etiology and/or prognosis) operate to help parents come to terms with reality and the decisions required of them as a result of that reality. The expiating function is similar, but the form and content of these conveniences and explanations change over time.

A final observation is that there seems to exist behind this history an almost universal capacity-based view of value. Newborns were not generally vested with value equal to older humans. Neither were they necessarily immediately given status or place within social organizations, either the family or society. Thus, it seems that newborns were perceived either to possess by nature or human assignment a provisionary value that, for sufficient reason, could be licitly overridden. Such a view of newborn value could be seen to prefigure recently proposed property-based theories of personhood that were reviewed in Chapter 5. These theories seem to articulate centuries-old intuitions and practices based upon them. Pediatrician William Silverman has noted that only within the past hundred years have the institutions of religion, law, and medicine sought to restrict parents from acting on these perceptions of relative value. Nevertheless, in Silverman's opinion, these efforts have been ''unsuccessful in obliterating the ancient view that distinguished between the death of a neonate and the loss of life of a self-conscious rational human being.''[44]

This is not to suggest that the death of a newborn, defective or normal, is not an occasion for grief. But in situations of conflict where the interests of a severely compromised newborn are compared to interests of others (for example, older healthy siblings), there seems to be relevant material differences between the newborn and others, almost universally perceived, such as to sanction the loss of the neonate in order to respect and preserve the interests of others. This overview of explanatory factors of infanticide suggests that proposals and actions to end the life of a defective newborn reasonably believed incapable of a minimal level of independence or personal existence deserve serious consideration. Parents who arrive at these conclusions may not be expressing a frivolous desire based on trivial reasons. They may, in fact, be expressing a considered judgment grounded in a moral consciousness and social history of long duration.

Killing and Letting Die: A Suspect Distinction

As has been seen, the distinction between active killing and mere letting die has played a significant role in the history of infanticide, both as a factor easing the psychological burden of guilt on the part of the infanticidal parents, and as a direct legal convenience to such parents. The influence of this distinction continues to be exerted in modern newborn nurseries and in courts.[45] Yet the distinction itself and its relevance to moral evaluations have come under increasingly convincing attack by philosophers and others concerned with questions of applied ethics. A survey of the most important of these attacks, together with an evaluation of the most capable rejoinders made by adherents of the distinction, will serve to establish the position that, in and of itself, the distinction between killing and letting die has no moral significance.

The killing/letting die distinction is an application, to cases involving death, of the more general distinction between actively violating a moral prohibition (e.g., do not kill) and merely omitting to perform a (possibly morally required) action (e.g., aid a person in peril). This general distinction can, in turn, be separated into a nonmoral and a moral component. The nonmoral component is the distinction, roughly, between doing and re-fraining.[46] Some philosophers have argued that the distinction between doing and refraining could never be formulated with sufficient precision to render it a reliable tool for moral evalua-tion.[47] Others have responded by offering modifications of the distinction that, arguably, extend its range of applicability to cover previously troublesome cases.[48] This dispute is mentioned only to set it aside.[49] Of greater concern for the present work is the question, What moral significance, if any, is possessed by the doing/refraining distinction, once it is granted for the sake of the argument that the distinction either is or could be formulated with sufficient precision to make it practically servicable? An answer to this question will come from an examination of the second—the *moral*—component of the general distinction between evil ac-tion and evil omission. That component can be formulated roughly in the following way: To act so as to bring about evil is morally more serious than to refrain from an action that would prevent a like evil.[50]

This idea has been repeatedly attacked in recent years, chiefly by philosophers with utilitarian tendencies. This is not surprising since, for a utilitarian, all that is relevant to moral evaluation, either of actions or of omissions, is the net balance of utility or net benefit attaching to resulting states of affairs. Whether those states of affairs result from action or from forebearance is deemed irrelevant where the total consequences are equivalent.[51]

Persons who have been persuaded by utilitarian arguments also have recognized that most people's moral intuitions conform to the idea that it is morally worse to kill than to let die. They therefore have seen that their denial of the acting/refraining dis-tinction could be strengthened if they could somehow explain away the doctrine's popular intuitive appeal. The general ap-proach to this end has been to admit, on the one hand, that many if not most instances of wrongful action *are* morally worse, all things considered, than correspondingly wrongful omissions, and to deny, on the other hand, that this difference in moral gravity is at all a result of the distinction between action and omission per se. It is then claimed that the difference in moral gravity, all things considered, between actions and omissions can be ex-plained by the fact that many if not most wrongful actions possess certain *other* wrong-making characteristics[52] that, though they *could* also be possessed by wrongful omissions, are most often confined to actions. That such other characteristics are usually confined to actions explains why actions are, on balance and all things considered, usually deemed morally worse than omissions with equally grave consequences. That such other characteristics *could* be possessed by omissions has been taken to show that, under appropriate circumstances, an omission and an action with equally grave consequences would have to be evaluated as morally equivalent, and thus that the general nonmoral distinction between action and omission has no moral significance in itself.[53]

Proponents of the acting/refraining distinction are unconvinced by consequentialist objections. They offer, however, and perhaps paradoxically, a consequentialist argument in its defense. For example, when applied to situations where a patient is expected to die, they fear "that permitting active killing for mercy will lead to more active killing for other reasons."[54] More generally, this is the fear that the rejection of the distinction will result in people coming to view wrongful actions as *no worse* than wrongful omissions, with the consequence that wrongful actions may proliferate to intolerable levels. As will be shown, the argument has little compelling force.

A more powerful version of the consequentialist defense takes the form of a dilemma. Once the distinction is rejected, people's attitudes could be changed in either of two ways: first, they might continue to have their present, seriously negative attitudes toward evil action, in which case the rejection of the distinction would entail that they would alter their attitudes toward evil omission so as to make the two sets of attitudes *equally seriously negative;* or second, they might continue to have their present, less seriously negative attitudes toward evil omissions, in which case the rejection of the distinction would entail that they would alter their attitudes toward evil action so as to make the two sets of attitudes *equally,* though *less seriously,* negative.[55]

If the former were to result, the argument maintains that this would place impossible demands on everyone. For example, once failure to send food to starving people in Africa came to be viewed at an equally grave moral level as the active killing of innocent persons, morality would demand great sacrifice on the part of those better off to assure that no one less well off went hungry. But since the number of unfortunate people who could benefit from the assistance of those better off is so great, it is likely that the sacrifice required by morality would be never ending and all consuming. Alternatively, if the latter were to result, the argument maintains that murder might become as commonplace as is the letting die of starving people in Africa. Yet the rejection of the distinction, according to this defense, entails that either consequence will occur. Hence, whichever results, the rejection has an unacceptable consequence, which shows that the distinction must be maintained as a principle guiding moral choice.

This is a weak argument for a number of reasons. The main defect of the dilemma is a logical failure. Rejecting the acting/refraining distinction amounts to a claim that one must view, for example, an act that stops a causal process that results in a good or evil outcome as morally equivalent to a failure to initiate a causal process, assuming one has power to do so, and thereby preventing a good or evil outcome.[56] In short, one's moral judgment about stopping an action and not starting it must be symmetrical, i.e., both are judged good or bad if the outcome in either case is the same. One consequence of this type of symmetrical moral judgment is the claim that "the characteristic of being an act of killing a person is no more [or less] serious a wrong-making characteristic than that of being an act of failing to save someone."[57] But it should be pointed out that it is *only* claims about the relative seriousness of wrong-making characteristics that are entailed by symmetrical moral judgments, or by the denial of the acting/refraining distinction. Nothing at all is implied about the relative seriousness of wrongful actions vis-à-vis wrongful omissions *all things* (i.e., all wrong-making characteristics) *considered*.

Consider the attitude changes described above. In both cases, the claim is made that rejection of the acting/refraining distinction would bring about changes in people's attitudes toward the relative seriousness of wrongful actions vis-à-vis wrongful omissions *all things considered*. Now, a claim is ambiguous. On one interpretation of the phrase "bring about" the claim amounts to the assertion that rejection of the distinction somehow logically entails attitude changes such as those already described. But this is clearly false, since rejection of the distinction and/or judging acts and omissions symmetrically only involves taking a stand on the relative seriousness of wrong-making characteristics, and need not logically imply anything about the relative seriousness of actions and omissions, all things considered.

On another interpretation of the phrase "bring about," the claim amounts to the assertion that, whether or not there is any *logical* connection between rejecting the distinction and the above attitude changes, people's attitudes would *in fact* be altered, either as in the former or as in the latter, if the distinction were widely rejected. That is, people would probably *mistakenly* alter their attitudes to view omissions that end in evil as negatively as evil deeds, or view evil actions less negatively than before but now equal with omissions, solely on the basis of their rejection of the acting/refraining distinction. This seems to be medical ethicist Robert Veatch's point when he asserts, "[I]f one of the features of active killing for mercy is that it might lead to active killing for other reasons because *in general people cannot adequately make a relevant moral distinction*, then that consequence might count against active killing for mercy" (emphasis added).[58]

One gets an inkling of the defectiveness of this line of reasoning by considering the following roughly similar argument: If people were allowed to own and drive automobiles bad consequences would result. People cannot be trusted to drive safely, and so many harmful accidents would result. Therefore, people should not be allowed to own and drive automobiles. The general form of both arguments is: If we put into people's hands certain otherwise perfectly legitimate things (automobiles or authority to judge acts and omissions symmetrically), they might make mistakes in the application of those things, with the result that harmful consequences would ensue. It would be better, then, to withhold the otherwise legitimate things than to provide the opportunity for such mistakes.

Two points are, in my opinion, decisive against this argument. First, what the consequentialist or slippery slope argument for the acting/refraining distinction is supposed to be establishing is the *validity* of the distinction as a principle guiding moral choice. But the argument does not establish the distinction's validity; rather, it merely points to possible undesirable results of the widespread rejection of it. Unless one is a rule-utilitarian, one would not accept this strategy as in any way testifying to the validity of the distinction. Second, the argument does not establish anything about the possible evil consequences of the distinction's rejection, which a similar argument could not establish with respect to any other moral principle. As Veatch admits, what worries him about the rejection of the acting/refraining distinction is the memory of how the principle of beneficent euthanasia was exploited by the Nazis in their eugenics program. What he apparently fails to note, however, is that the Nazis did not simply make a *mistake* about the proper bounds of beneficent euthanasia. Instead, they exploited an existing and perhaps morally defensible policy according to the demands of a previously formulated political agenda.

Surely *any* existing moral or legal principle is subject to intentional misuse by persons seeking to implement a malevolent agenda. For example, even highly regarded American principles of economic and political justice could be twisted so as to systematically exclude whole groups from their aegis, resulting in great harm to the groups affected. That such discrimination existed here in the past gives ample reason to believe that it could happen again in the future. And for that reason we do not call into question the principles of justice themselves. Rather, we remain vigilant and erect elaborate safeguards to assure that those principles will not be so abused. Similarly, the experience of eugenics in Nazi Germany should not cause us to question the appropriateness of the rejection of the acting/refraining distinction if that principle is found wanting, as it has been. Procedures or other mechanisms of oversight could be established to limit mistakes, misuses, or malevolent applications of a rejection of the acting/refraining distinction; that is, safeguards against otherwise avoidable deaths would be proper. For example, licensing is an effort to establish a minimal degree of competency for driving automobiles. In the realm of health care, second opinions or confirming tests certifying that an incompetent patient is irretrievably near death might be required before life-supports are not initiated or are withdrawn, or before death is induced.

In addition to procedures or mechanisms, massive public programs could be undertaken to educate people about when it is appropriate to hasten death given the invalidity of the acting/refraining distinction as a reason not to do so. These activities could be more efficient and effective overall in safeguarding patients than procedures or laws. Civil rights legislation was hoped to lessen injustices done to blacks. But changed public attitudes toward blacks, attitudes less dominated by ignorance and prejudice, have probably done more than the law to bring about their just treatment. In the same way, public awareness that the moral symmetry of killing and letting die applies most properly in cases where a patient's death cannot be avoided, or where death is reasonably judged better for the patient than prolonged life, may be a more effective and efficient safeguard than procedures or laws.

To conclude, the arguments in favor of the acting/refraining distinction fail whether interpreted as expressing a *logical*, or merely a probable *psychological*, connection between its widespread rejection and attitudinal changes that might result in unwanted consequences. I do not claim to have shown the acting/refraining distinction to be false. What I claim is that, given the skepticism toward the distinction among philosophers, the burden of proof regarding this principle rests squarely on its defenders. Unless convincing arguments are generated in defense of the alleged distinction, we should remain agnostic on the issue of its validity. Yet life and death decisions regarding severely defective newborns must be made. These decisions ought to be based on sound moral and medical principles. So long as the jury is out on the acting/refraining distinction, other moral and medical principles can lead us to the conclusion that, in many cases, actively promoting the death of a severely defective newborn is no worse—and, in fact, is often better—all things considered, than letting the newborn die. We seem more prepared to allow the latter, and on the basis of the analysis here, an uncertain principle (that an action which results in evil is more morally wrong than an omission which results in evil) ought not stand in our way of doing the former.[59] In these instances, mercifully ending life is not morally wrong. It can be morally right.

Selective Infanticide: Regrettable but Acceptable

We return in this concluding section to the question with which this chapter began: May neonates who will never attain a personal existence, never experience life as a net value, and/or never achieve a minimal level of independence be mercifully terminated? This question has been of interest to philosophers as shown in the discussion of the alleged moral distinction between killing and letting die or acting and refraining from action. Parents of severely defective neonates and the neonatal medical team, however, consider this question in a context in which real lives are at stake and the decisions that are made will result in real consequences.

John Freeman, an expert in the treatment of spina bifida, expresses the dilemma as follows: "Is it moral to encourage the survival of a child who will be a paraplegic, incontinent, and will require multiple surgical procedures for hydrocephalus, orthopedic deformity, and bladder dysfunction? . . . If we elect *not* to treat a child, what becomes of him? Is he to be fed and watered while the physician waits for him to develop meningitis? Is he to be sedated and fed inadequately so that he dies slowly of starvation without making too much noise? Or are we to kill him overtly? Or covertly? Actively rather than passively?"[60] Later in the same article Freeman admits, "active euthanasia might be the most humane course for the *most severely* affected infants, but it is illegal. 'Passive euthanasia' is legal, but is hardly humane." He continues, that "until active euthanasia for the most severely affected children becomes socially acceptable to society, we must opt for vigorous treatment, to make these children and their families as intact as we are able."[61]

Englishman John Lorber, a specialist in the newborn who does not favor life-extending treatment for all cases of spina bifida, considered euthanasia "fully logical" and a "humane way" of dealing with newborns who, if treated, will survive with life-disvaluing handicaps.[62] Raymond Duff and A. G. M. Campbell are neonatologists who call for a change in the law to permit causing the deaths of selected newborns as a means of liberating the infant from pointless, dehumanizing treatment.[63] Parents and physicians should be allowed to make these decisions on the basis of available medical evidence and according to their defensible moral vision. Duff and Campbell conclude, "In view of the complexities of human experience and human tragedy and the difficulties and conflicts in deciding the proper use of medical technology, this approach to the problem of life and death control seems to make sense."[64] I agree.

Decisions to accept the deaths of these imperiled and/or severely debilitated infants are characteristically sorrowful. The present practice is to orchestrate their deaths under the guise of allowing nature to take its course. This procedure can result in a prolonged, painful death for the infant and extended suffering for the community of the dying infant. Unintended and unnecessary costs (broadly understood) can accompany this presumably sensitive practice. But in cases in which the evils of pain, suffering, and death are chosen among, effecting the deaths of

these infants is a morally valid, and at times preferable, alternative to the current practice. This is an alternative that requires a
delicate balance of mercy, courage, and wisdom. It can be a just
and beneficent response to a tragic situation requiring the most
compassionate and dignified expression of the moral community.[65]

For some infants, death is a morally reasonable end for parents and neonatologists to seek. Providing a merciful death to
these carefully selected infants is morally licit. It is permissible
from a moral point of view (not legal) to bring about the most
peaceable and aesthetic death possible, both for the infant and
for those intimately related to it. In a society that sanctions the
termination of fetal life for reasons of defect, it is illogical to deny
this option to parents with regard to similarly situated newborns.
The birth canal, and the passage of developing human life through
it, is of no moral significance in these cases. Parents, in these tragic
circumstances, should be free from moral blame if they reasonably decide that death, all things considered, is in the best interest
of this newborn infant or indicated because the costs of prolonging its life are found sufficient to defeat customary duties of beneficence toward it. Neonatologists, as a sustaining presence,
should be free to cooperate, to the extent their professional and
moral commitments will permit, with parents to bring about a
merciful end to a tragic sequence of events. Reason and moral
argument surely warrant such a conclusion. But common sense,
too, can lead to a similar judgment.

Recall the case of the infant born with a skin condition similar
to third-degree burns over almost all of its body for which there
was no cure. The baby's mother was young, unwed, and indigent. Providing basic nursing care caused tearing away of the
skin. The infant could not be fed orally because of blistering in
the mouth and throat. Any movement of the infant seemed to
cause it pain. Even with intensive care its life expectancy, at most,
was believed to be days. Wouldn't it have been reasonable, merciful, and justifiable to have shortened the baby's dying by an
intended, direct action? Wouldn't such an action chosen by the
parents[66] and acceptable to the neonatologists be beneficent and
just? Couldn't such an action represent a choice for a lesser evil?
My answer in each instance is yes. In cases relevantly like this,
it is not immoral or morally wrong to intend and effect a merciful
end to a life that, all things considered, will be meaningless to

the one who lives it and an unwarranted burden for others to support.

The exposition of the practice of infanticide with which this chapter began shows that people throughout almost all of history have understood that under certain circumstances a hastened death for a newborn is an acceptable means of preserving certain other goods that otherwise would be lost as a result of the continued life of particular newborn infants. In those instances today in which a baby is born with a disease or defect such that it can be judged reasonably to foreclose (1) the attainment of capacities for minimal independence, (2) the attainment of capacities sufficient for personhood, (3) whose survival would impose a burden on the infant such as to render life a net disvalue, or (4) whose severely impaired survival would impose upon others an unreasonable, grave, disproportionate, or incommensurate burden, a decision that intends death for the newborn could be morally justified. When death for a newborn is a morally justifiable intention and outcome, it is as morally licit to bring about this end by merciful means as it would be to stand aside while death occurs by so-called natural means. The moral status of a human neonate is such that it is not a person in the strict sense. It is not capable of self-determination. It is not a bearer of rights and duties, including unlimited duties of beneficence and rights to forebearance. Human neonates, because of the role they have in the moral community, are persons only in a social sense. Some people *may* impute personhood to them and regard them as if they are persons, but their capacities are as yet undeveloped to the degree sufficient for personhood in a strict moral sense. Accordingly, customary rights to forebearance (i.e., not to be killed against their consent) are not violated when a merciful and aesthetic death is provided for those neonates who meet at least one of the four conditions listed above.

There can be no doubt that neonatology is a hotbed of medical, moral, and legal debate. Often the choice available to individuals responsible for the care of these infants is limited to a choice among disvalued ends or evils. No one is happy that, at times, these are the only options available. However, not to decide for and act in a manner that pursues the least evil may result unnecessarily in a greater evil. Choosing among evils requires wisdom and courage. We need wisdom to select properly among means and ends. We need courage to act on wise choices. When faced with unfortunate situations that demand "sound and se-rene judgment regarding the conduct of life"[67] may we have the courage to act, even if others believe that we ought not.

The controversies regarding the medical care of severely dis-eased or defective newborns have not escaped the attention of makers of public policy and officials of the law. Developments at this level of discussion will be surveyed in the next chapter, where we shall also consider how recent policy initiatives and the law relate to the perspectives and conclusions offered in this volume.

7

Parental Authority and Public Policy

Developments in obstetric and neonatal medicine have moved the locus of delivery and newborn care out of the home and into the hospital. This shift has helped to make private reproductive tragedies the pawns of the ideological and political struggle over the value of human life. As particular infants and decisions regarding their care are publicized more and more, decisions that accept and/or intend the deaths of certain infants have aroused public concern, provoked efforts to foreclose certain options, and generated procedural proposals designed to certify the propriety of treatment choices. The interest of the public or society in this sort of matter is routinely expressed through law, either in its legislative, judicial, or regulatory form. There has been activity at the federal level on all three fronts aimed at limiting parental authority and discretion with regard to the medical management of severely defective or diseased infants.

The legal survey in Chapter 2 showed a presumption for parental autonomy and family privacy in matters regarding the care and nurture of children. It was observed that there is a marked reluctance in the law to intervene in family life but that the state would do so for sufficient reason. Despite a presumption of parental competency, the state was seen to have a vaguely defined interest in protecting children, including newborn infants, from parental abuse and neglect. This vaguely defined interest is often in contention with the state's interest in protecting parental authority and family privacy, especially in areas such as newborn medicine where diverse licit values have a dominant role in fashioning decisions and determining actions that are perceived to impact negatively on children. When the state perceives that a child or class of children is unreasonably endangered, it can act to protect its interest through its police and *parens patriae* powers.

The propensity of government, especially at the federal level, to intervene in the arena of medical decision making for severely impaired neonates has increased significantly since April 1982. The apparent reasons for this effort to limit and/or usurp parental authority in this realm and the forms that governmental actions have taken are the subjects of this final chapter. More specifically, the apparent precipitating events involving treatment decisions for imperiled newborns and the federal responses to them will be surveyed and analyzed. This review will include an examination of regulatory and judicial activity associated with the so-called Baby Doe rules, and a report on the Federal Child Abuse Amendments of 1984, which refer to the medical care of disabled infants. These activities will be evaluated and found overall to reflect misperceptions of the role of the state in these tragic circumstances, of the moral status of the newborn, and of enforceable duties of beneficence. In addition, these efforts to reshape public policy will be found not to constitute a significant improvement over current customary practices of relying primarily on parental and medical judgments regarding these complex and perplexing cases.

Regulatory and Judicial Proceedings

The genesis of recent federal involvement in deciding the medical care of newborns with severe diseases or defects was a case in Bloomington, Indiana, involving an infant born with Down syndrome and a tracheoesophageal fistula. This male infant was born April 9, 1982, to a thirty-one-year-old woman who had two healthy children at home. The social and financial circumstances of the parents are not known. Neither is it known what religious beliefs the parents held, if any. At birth Baby Doe, as he became known during the course of court proceedings, was limp and cyanotic, had a heart rate of less than 100, and Apgar scores of 5 and 7 at one minute and five minutes, respectively. Baby Doe weighed almost 6 pounds (2,722 grams) at birth. Initial diagnoses of Down syndrome and tracheoesophageal fistula were made following delivery. Chest X-rays revealed an enlarged heart that, together with other signs, led to a diagnosis of possible aortic coartation. The parents, following consultation with physicians, refused surgery that would have repaired the fistula, and enabled the infant to be fed orally. Medicines for pain and restlessness were given.

On April 10, one day after the birth of Baby Doe, the hospital's attorney asked the County Circuit Court to hear the case. Several physicians apparently testified that the child should be transferred to another hospital and the corrective surgery ordered despite the parents' decision to the contrary. The judge refused to issue the requested order, accepting the parents' and attending physician's judgment that a Down syndrome child would never have a "minimally acceptable quality of life." Further, the court held that the parents, given their knowledge of the contrasting medical opinions, "have the right to choose a medically recommended course of treatment for their child in the present circumstances." The court ordered the hospital to allow the treatment agreed upon by the parents and attending physician. Further legal efforts to mandate corrective surgery were unsuccessful.[1] Six days after Baby Doe's birth, he died.

Notice to Health Care Providers, May 18, 1982

On April 30, 1982, fifteen days following the death of Baby Doe, President Ronald Reagan notified the secretary of the Department of Health and Human Services that federal law prohibits discrimination against handicapped individuals. Acting on the president's concern, Betty Lou Dotson, director of the Office for Civil Rights, issued, on May 18, 1982, a "Notice to Health Care Providers." Citing Section 504 of the Rehabilitation Act of 1973,[2] she reminded providers of health care that "it is unlawful for a recipient of Federal financial assistance to withhold from a handicapped infant nutritional sustenance or medical or surgical treatment required to correct a life-threatening condition, if: (1) the withholding is based on the fact that the infant is handicapped; and (2) the handicap does not render the treatment or nutritional sustenance medically contraindicated."[3] Down syndrome, one impairment of Baby Doe, was specifically identified as a handicapping condition that would effectively bring all Down patients within the provisions of the Notice.

The Department of Health and Human Services acknowledged that hospitals do not have full control over the treatments provided to handicapped patients, particularly in those instances, such as Baby Doe, where "parental consent has been refused." Nevertheless, hospitals were warned not to "aid or perpetuate discrimination by significantly assisting the discriminatory actions of another person or organization." As an incentive for care providers to comply with the provisions of the Notice, they were advised that failure to conform their practices and policies could result in "possible termination of Federal assistance," i.e., payment for services through federal programs.

The reaction of hospitals, physicians, and others to the Notice was not uniformly enthusiastic. A response by pediatrician Norman Fost was fairly typical. Fost's complaints focused on two substantive issues related to language within the Notice. From a pediatrician's perspective, Fost noted that "it is not clear if or why a handicap can *never* be a justification for withholding treatment."[4] Suppose, Fost says, that a newborn is essentially like Karen Quinlan, "permanently unable to engage in social interactions," and who also has no kidneys. Renal dialysis could prolong such an infant's life but, Fost asks, what is the point or justification of doing so. Presumably, the provisions of the Notice would require dialysis since there would not be a medical contraindication to doing so. But, he explains, the nature and extent of the infant's handicap, contrary to the Notice, would be a moral and legal reason to withhold dialysis. The child would not "experience any benefit of the treatment," due to a handicap that is so severe "as to make further life, and therefore further treatment, not in [its] . . . interest."[5]

Fost thinks that the justification for nontreatment is found in the second clause of the Notice, which requires treatment *unless* "the handicap makes treatment medically contraindicated." But the wording of this exemption is considered "vague" and "unintelligible." As such, it is the subject of his second substantive complaint. The meaning of "medical contraindication" is not clear. If the Notice essentially permits physicians to use "good judgment" in caring for patients, then, according to Fost, the Notice is not needed.[6] Fost speculates that the government had more in mind than this. However, he is unable to determine exactly what is intended from the wording of the Notice. It seems to say that a handicap is not *in some cases* a valid reason to withhold life-sustaining treatment. But according to Fost, the "fundamental defect of Section 504 [as interpreted in the Notice] is its failure to distinguish between handicaps that justify nontreatment and those which do not."[7] The intent of the orders regarding provider practices and policies is clearer but, in Fost's opinion, could result in the discharge of infants from hospitals only to receive less care than they would have otherwise.[8]

Interim Final Rule, March 7, 1983

As controversial as the Notice was, it provoked only a brushfire of protest compared to the firestorm of debate generated by an "interim final rule" issued by the secretary of the Department of Health and Human Services, on March 7, 1983, regarding "Non-discrimination on the Basis of Handicap."[9] This interim final rule built upon the described "substantive obligations of health care providers" contained in the Notice of May 18, 1982. Designated to become effective on March 22, 1983, fifteen days following their issuance, the interim final rule "modifie[d] existing regulations to meet the exigent needs that can arise when a handicapped infant is discriminatorily denied food or other medical care." The regulatory modifications were designed "to allow timely reporting of violations, expeditious investigation, and immediate enforcement action when necessary to protect a handicapped infant whose life is endangered by discrimination in a program or activity receiving Federal financial assistance."[10] The rules state that the secretary intended to rely upon and work with state and local agencies that are customarily responsible for the protection of infants. However, the specific provisions of the rules indicate clearly that the federal government was prepared to assume a role of oversight that it never before had taken.

The rule had three provisions. First, it required recipient providers to post and keep posted "in a conspicuous place in each delivery ward, each maternity ward, each pediatric ward, and each nursery, including each intensive care nursery" a notice stating *"Discriminatory Failure to Feed and Care for Handicapped Infants in This Facility is Prohibited by Federal Law."* The text of the notice referred to Section 504 of the Rehabilitation Act of 1973 for authorization and proceeded to advise "Any person having knowledge that a handicapped infant is being discriminatorily denied food or customary medical care should immediately contact: Handicapped Infant Hotline. . . . "[11] A toll-free number to be answered twenty-four hours a day followed. Whistle-blowers were told that they additionally or alternately could contact the state child protection agency, that retaliation or intimidation toward a reporter was prohibited by federal law, and that a caller's identity would be kept confidential. The posted notice ended with an announcement that "Failure to feed and care for infants may also violate the criminal and civil laws of your State."[12]

The rule's second provision created a narrow exception to the ten-day delay between the time the secretary finds that a recipient has failed to comply with existing regulations and legal action to effect compliance. This exception was believed necessary because "immediate remedial action is necessary to protect the life or health of a handicapped individual. . . . being denied food or other necessary medical care."[13] Similarly, the third provision required immediate access to records and facilities by federal investigators "when, in the judgment of the responsible Department official, immediate access is necessary to protect the life or health of a handicapped individual."[14]

These new regulations are explained by the secretary as necessary to protect handicapped infants from discrimination and to save their lives. While noting that the federal government intended to notify state child protective agencies of received complaints, the secretary reserved the right to take direct federal action necessary to save the life of a handicapped child subjected to discrimination or to protect a complainant. All of these actions indicative of an emergency situation were taken even though the secretary admited, that "The full extent of discriminatory and life-threatening practices toward handicapped infants is not yet known, but the Secretary believes that for even a single infant to die due to lack of an adequate notice and complaint procedure is unacceptable."[15]

A coalition of plaintiffs—consisting of the American Academy of Pediatrics, National Association of Children's Hospitals and Related Institutions, and Children's Hospital National Medical Center—sued the secretary of the Department of Health and Human Services, Margaret M. Heckler, in the United States District Court, District of Columbia, challenging the validity of the "interim final rule," then popularly known as the "Baby Doe" rules. Judge Gesell, in an opinion dated April 14, 1983, set aside the regulations on procedural grounds. The court observed that the Administrative Procedure Act "was designed to curb bureaucratic actions taken without consultation and notice to persons affected" and that the regulation was an "offense" to the established precepts of that Act "to a remarkable extent."[16] Lacking a rational and factual basis, Judge Gesell found the rule "invalid as an arbitrary and capricious agency action. . . . "[17] In addition, the rule was determined invalid due to the secretary's failure to comply with established procedures of public notice or to delay their effective date for thirty days as required by the Administrative Procedure Act.[18]

In expanding on his first finding, Judge Gesell observed that the secretary gave no consideration whatsoever to the potentially disruptive effects of the implementation of the rule. The prospect of "the sudden descent of 'Baby Doe' squads on the scene, monopolizing physician and nurse time and making hospital charts and records unavailable during treatment," in the judge's opinion, "can hardly be presumed to produce higher quality care for the infant."[19] Turning to the text of the rule which indicated that failure to provide customary medical care to a handicapped infant is a violation of federal law, on the basis of evidence presented at trial, Judge Gesell determined that *"there is no customary standard of care* for the treatment of severely defective newborns. The regulation thus purports to set up an enforcement mechanism without defining the violation, and is virtually without meaning beyond its intrinsic *in terrorem* effect" (emphasis added).[20]

The opinion further states that the "defendant's [HHS] counsel acknowledged in argument, the regulation is intended, among other things, to change the course of medical decision-making in these cases by eliminating the parents' right to refuse to consent to life-sustaining treatment of their defective newborn."[21] Judge Gesell was not very sympathetic to this objective. He writes,

> The Secretary did not appear to give the slightest consideration to the advantages and disadvantages of relying on the *wishes of the parents* who, knowing the setting in which the child may be raised, in many ways are in the *best position to evaluate the infant's best interest*. Ignoring parental preferences again may increase the risk that parents will withdraw the infant from hospital care entirely, and the long-term interests of physically disabled new-

borns may be affected by thrusting the child into situations where
economic and marital effects on the family as a whole are so
adverse that the effort to preserve an unwanted child may require concurrent attention to procedures for adoption or other
placement.

   None of these sensitive considerations touching so intimately
on the *quality of the infant's expected life* were even tentatively
noted. No attempt was made to address the issue of whether
termination of painful, intrusive medical treatment *might be appropriate* where an infant's clear prognosis is death within days
or months or to specify the level of appropriate care in such futile
cases. [Emphasis added][22]

These sentiments and concerns are consistent with the emphasis
placed on parental autonomy and responsibility in this volume.
As is evident from the judge's remarks, there is legal precedent
for a presumption of parental authority and for taking quality-of-
life factors into consideration as decisions regarding the best interests of defective newborns are made.

Proposed Rules, July 5, 1983

Judge Gesell's ruling invalidating the "Baby Doe" rules, however, is not the end of the regulatory story. Not to be denied, and
taking notice of the procedural defects relied upon by Judge Gesell, the Department issued on July 5, 1983, proposed rules regarding "Nondiscrimination on the Basis of Handicap Relating to
Health Care for Handicapped Infants."[23] The proposed rule was
in substantive agreement with the one invalidated by Judge Gesell. However, to overcome the procedural defects, comments regarding the proposed rules were invited to be received by
September 6, 1983, sixty days following issuance. Further, the Department attempted to establish in the preamble a rationale and
factual basis for the rules citing a report of a Presidential Commission, articles published in medical journals describing nontreatment practices, several isolated but publicized cases, and
surveys of medical opinion regarding the medical management
of defective newborns.

   The rules of July 5, 1983, limited posting notices to locations
visible to health care personnel rather than to the general public.
The text was changed slightly. The only substantive change re-

quired state child protection agencies within sixty days following the effective date of the proposed rules to establish methods and procedures to require reporting of suspected instances of medical neglect, to facilitate prompt investigation of reports, to take protective action when found necessary, and to notify the Department's Office for Civil Rights of their findings and actions in each case.[24] This addition, which puts investigation and enforcement primarily within state agencies, seems to evidence the federal government's lack of expertise to investigate child abuse complaints.[25]

The same standard of customary medical care questioned by Judge Gesell was retained in the second draft of the now-proposed rule. In an effort to provide content to this standard and to clarify the applicability of Section 504 with regard to handicapped infants, explanatory comments are provided in an appendix. In short, Section 504 is said to be an "equal treatment, nondiscrimination standard"[26] that effectively forbids unequal treatment on the basis of handicap in a manner similar to Title VI of the Civil Rights Act, which forbids unequal treatment on the basis of race. With regard to customary medical care, the Department states that handicapped infants cannot be denied, solely by reason of their handicap, benefits and services that "are appropriate, in the exercise of *reasonable medical judgment*, to the circumstance of the particular handicapped infant."[27] The explanatory comments disclaim a desire to "intrude upon legitimate medical opinion" or to mandate treatment "contrary to reasonable medical judgment—i.e., 'medically contraindicated.'"[28] However, the text observes that all judgments made by physicians are not strictly "medical" judgments of the prospective net benefits of possible treatments or interventions. Section 504, according to the appendix, would not extend to treatment of "dubious medical benefit to the patient or if the patient could not long survive even with the treatment, reasonable medical judgment could withhold the treatment"[29] without violating the law. Neither are "impossible," "futile," or "merely" death-prolonging interventions within the scope of Section 504.

Several examples are provided to differentiate cases and treatments. An anencephalic infant would not require life-prolonging efforts since "on the basis of the legitimate medical judgment . . . the child would die imminently even with treatment. The decision to withhold treatment," it is explained, "is therefore not

based on handicap. . . . " An extremely low birth weight infant
might be denied life-sustaining care "if the decision is based on
a reasonable medical judgment concerning improbability of success in a course of treatment, or risks and potential harm in the
course of treatment." Nevertheless, feeding, watering, and routine nursing care are required as matters of "human dignity."
Failure to perform these functions are construed to violate Section
504. The class of infants and handicaps that qualify for Section
504 protection are described as "those handicapped infants . . .
who would live if given treatment for a life-threatening congenital
anomaly . . . " and who have treatment withheld on the basis of
a handicap "such as mental retardation, blindness, paralysis,
deafness, or lack of limbs," rather than nontreatment on the basis
of medical judgment free from any assessment of the worthiness
of the patient for treatment. Examples of discriminatory withholding of treatment include such infants as Baby Doe (Down syndrome accompanied by operable defects), infants with spina bifida
accompanied by correctable anomalies the treatment of which is
not medically considered futile or of questionable net benefit, and
infants who otherwise would be treated except for an actual or
potential handicap.[30]

These examples surely were hoped to be helpful explanations
of the intent, scope, and application of the proposed rule. It
should be observed, however, that the effort failed. Certain anencephalic babies can, in fact, live for an extended time with appropriate medical and nursing support—though the existence is
vegetative. Thus, it appears that the rule either covertly or im-
plicitly accepts some form of quality-of-life criteria in determining
the value of life to some handicapped infants, but not others.
Similarly, the level of low birth weight below which efforts to rescue are not required is not specified—some infants weighing little
more than $17\frac{1}{2}$ ounces (500 grams) at birth seem able to, at least,
survive with intensive care. Neither does the explanation specify
the degree of "improbability" nor the criteria for "success" below or without which nontreatment is considered nondiscrimi-
natory. Finally, in light of the discussion in Chapter 6, it could be
questioned whether the provision of food and water to an infant
whose death is accepted or intended is not more responsive to
the possible psychological discomfort of bystanders than required
by moral reasoning.

The explanations and examples contained in the appendix, together with these brief responses illustrate how difficult and problematic is any effort to codify customary medical care. The Department's recognition of this fact may be revealed by the repeated references to "legitimate medical judgment" to distinguish treatments and cases. If the Department was prepared, in fact, to defer to "legitimate medical opinion," then the conclusion of attorneys Angela Holder[31] and George Annas[32] that the proposed rules essentially restated existing standards of treatment and provisions for state enforcement of failures to observe the law, seems accurate.

The secretary had invited responses from interested parties regarding the proposed rules.[33] Comments from the American Academy of Pediatrics (AAP) were quite extensive and presumably partially persuasive, since some of their concerns are accommodated by revisions in the final rule. The AAP worried that the proposed rules would not remedy the perceived problem.[34] They noted that none of the investigations conducted prior to the invalidation of the original interim final rule revealed any impropriety. Further, the AAP worried that the provisions and procedures of the proposed rules were potentially harmful to critically ill infants. Reports were published that seem to substantiate this concern.[35]

An official policy statement,[36] included in the AAP response, noted the "impossibility" of defining clinical criteria for withholding treatment.[37] Stating that "the pediatrician's primary obligation is to the child" whose interests must be served if life-sustaining treatment is withheld or withdrawn, the AAP acknowledged that knowing the interests of the patient can be difficult. To enrich the process of this sort of life-and-death decision making, the policy statement recommended a consultation procedure involving a bioethics review committee, the structure and function of which would be consistent with a similar recommendation by the President's Commission for the Study of Ethical Problems in Medicine.[38]

The AAP observed that "[a]n institutional ethics committee will not be a panacea for making ethically correct decisions, but it should increase the probability that such decisions are informed and consistent with the broadest moral values of our society."[39] These committees, as envisaged by the AAP and others, were proposed to serve three functions: "(1) To develop hospital policies and guidelines for management of specific types of diagnoses; (2) to monitor adherence through retrospective record review; and (3) to review, on an emergency basis, specific cases when the withholding of life-sustaining treatment is being considered. When the committee disagreed with a parental or physician decision to withhold treatment, the case would be referred to the appropriate court or child protective agency, and treatment would be continued pending a decision."[40]

Final Rule, January 12, 1984

The final rules issued by HHS on January 12, 1984,[41] responded to several objections, most notably some dealing with the informational notice, the standard to guide treatment decisions, and recommendations for the establishment and operation of an Infant Care Review Committee. Despite substantive objections, the Department maintained its basic position in the final rules.

The informational notice was retitled "Principles of Treatment of Disabled Infants." It states that "nourishment and medically beneficial treatment (as determined with respect for reasonable medical judgments) should not be withheld from handicapped infants solely on the basis of their present or anticipated mental or physical impairments."[42] It should be noted that the standard to guide treatment decisions of "customary care" in the proposed rules was changed to "medically beneficial treatment" in the final rule. Futile or death-prolonging interventions are not considered medically beneficial. "Reasonable medical judgment" determines medical benefit and will not be overridden. Words changed but specificity and clarity were not increased. An almost unqualified bias to prolong life where possible, without regard to any quality-of-life considerations or parental wishes, is maintained.

The new rules incorporated the suggestion to utilize a committee review process but failed to mandate their establishment. Designated an Infant Care Review Committee (ICRC), it is "to assist the health care provider in the development of standards, policies and procedures for providing treatment to handicapped infants and in making decisions concerning medically beneficial treatment in specific cases."[43] By calling these committees Infant *Care*, not Infant *Bioethical*, Review Committees, an apparent steadfast intention to remove or, at least, minimize moral, value, and quality-of-life factors in making treatment decisions is betrayed. This point is underscored by the designation of "medical benefit" as the sole standard by which treatment decisions are to be made. Consideration of an infant's present or future handicap, availability of community resources, and impact on family or society are specifically excluded as relevant considerations. Where there is doubt concerning benefit, the rules establish a presumption in favor of treatment.[44] When parental decisions do not conform to this standard, hospitals are required to involve a state child protection agency or seek judicial review. Federal investigative procedures are revised to require consultation with local authorities and to lessen their potentially disruptive effect. In short, from the issuance of the "Notice to Health Care Providers" on May 18, 1982, to the final rules of January 12, 1984, very little of substance changed even though an extensive professional, scholarly, and public debate occurred in the interim.

Judicial Invalidation, February 23, 1984

But this is not the end of the story. While the final rules were being prepared an infant referred to as "Baby Jane Doe" was born on October 11, 1983, with "myelomeningocele, commonly known as spina bifida, a condition in which the spinal cord and membranes that envelop it are exposed; microcephaly, an abnormally small head; and hydrocephalus, a condition characterized by an accumulation of fluid in the cranial vault. In addition, she exhibited a 'weak face,' which prevents the infant from closing her eyes or making a full suck with her tongue; a malformed brain stem; upper extremity spasticity; and a thumb entirely within her fist."[45] The parents, after consultation with medical and religious advisors, refused permission for surgeries to close the opening in her spine and to drain fluids from the head. Neither procedure was likely to prolong her life or improve her disabling conditions. Instead, the parents authorized conservative care including feeding, antibiotics, and changing of dressings.

Lawrence Washburn, a right-to-life lawyer in Vermont, acting on a tip, brought suit in New York before Judge Melvyn Tanenbaum to order surgery for Baby Jane Doe. Judge Tanenbaum, who accepted the Right-to-Life party nomination for his candidacy in 1982, appointed William E. Weber as guardian *ad litem* to represent the infant at a hearing on October 20, 1983. Judge Tanenbaum "ruled the infant in need of immediate surgery to preserve her life and authorized Weber to consent to it."[46] Baby Jane Doe's parents appealed this ruling the next day. The Appellate Division reversed the trial court, finding the parents' decision consistent with the infant's best interests, thus negating the basis for judicial intervention. On appeal, the state's highest court, the Court of Appeals, used strong language in its opinion of October 28 affirming the Appellate Division's ruling, but for a different reason.

The Court of Appeals dismissed the suit on procedural grounds, noting that Washburn was without standing to initiate an action. Allegations of the sort brought by Washburn, according to state law, must be originated by a child protection agency or by someone authorized by a court to do so. Further, the law requires an investigation by the state child protection agency to determine if court proceedings are warranted. Since statutory provisions had not been followed the parents' decision was upheld. The court reasoned that to permit unrelated persons to initiate this sort of action apart from statutory provisions "would catapult him [a guardian or other plaintiff] into the very heart of a family circle, there to challenge the most private and most precious responsibility vested in the parents for the care and nurture of their children—and at the very least to force the parents to incur the not inconsiderable expenses of extended litigation."[47] The court called some of the activities and proceedings of the people seeking to displace the parents' responsibility in this matter "unusual," "offensive," and "distressing."

Meanwhile, the Department of Health and Human Services was getting involved. Acting on a hotline complaint, the Department asked the New York Child Protective Services to investigate the case of Baby Jane Doe. The agency reported no cause for intervention on November 7, 1983. Somehow, however, the medical records of Baby Jane Doe through October 19 were obtained and reviewed by U.S. Surgeon General C. Everett Koop. Koop was unable to determine if treatment had been denied on the basis of handicap without being able to review current medical records. These records were sought from University Hospital under authority of Section 504 of the Rehabilitation Act of 1973. The hospital refused and HHS brought suit in the U.S. District Court, Eastern District of New York, to obtain the medical records. In an opinion dated November 17, 1983, District Judge Wexler declined to order the hospital to release Baby Jane Doe's medical records.

Judge Wexler determined that the hospital had not discriminated against the infant. Failure to perform the surgical procedures at issue was due to a lack of parental consent, not a refusal by the hospital. Accordingly, the hospital was not in violation of Section 504. Judge Wexler described the parents' refusal "a reasonable one based on due consideration of the medical options available and on a genuine concern for the best interests of the child,"[48] a finding identical with medical opinion, the State Child Protection Service, the Appellate Division of the Supreme Court of New York, and the Court of Appeals of the State of New York.

Judge Wexler's opinion was appealed by the government in the United States Court of Appeals for the Second Circuit.[49] The Appeals Court focused on the issue of whether Section 504 authorized this type of investigation by the Department of HHS. Based on a review of the regulatory history of Section 504 of the Rehabilitation Act, the court determined that the Department's "current view of the scope of the statute is flatly at odds with the position originally taken by HEW."[50] Further, the legislative history of the Act was found not to support the government's claim that its scope included medical treatments of the type necessitated by Baby Jane Doe:

> The government has taken an oversimplified view of the medical decision-making process. Where the handicapping condition is related to the condition(s) to be treated, it will rarely, if ever, be possible to say with certainty that a particular decision was discriminatory. . . . Beyond the fact that no two cases are likely to be the same, it would invariably require lengthy litigation primarily involving conflicting expert testimony to determine whether a decision to treat, or not to treat, or to litigate or not to litigate, was based on a "bona fide medical judgment," however that phrase might be defined.[51]

Absent a clearer directive from Congress, the court refused to authorize Baby-Jane-Doe-type investigations. In short, the government was found not to have authority to involve itself in treatment decisions involving defective newborns. A subsequent U.S. District Court decision followed the Appeals Court and ruled the "Baby Doe Rules" "invalid" and "unlawful," and set them aside for lack of statutory authority.[52] The U.S. Supreme Court has agreed to decide whether the federal government has authority under Sec. 504 of the Rehabilitation Act to intervene in the care of severely impaired newborns. At the time of this writing, the

Court has not heard arguments or issued an opinion on this appeal by the Reagan Administration.

One is tempted to conclude that these several regulatory and judicial actions were pointless and ill-advised in light of the failure thus far of the government to have its way. Such a judgment, however, would be too harsh. These proceedings generated a sustained and critical discussion of substantive issues regarding the medical care of defective newborns. Questions of who decides and the proper bases of decisions were addressed, though often in a partisan fashion. The complex and perplexing character of these unfortunate situations were publicly aired. Media coverage of the controversy brought profound moral quandaries to the attention of the public. Whether, in the final analysis, these proceedings have helped to establish any form of consensus cannot be known. However, the regulatory and judicial story regarding treatment decisions for defective newborns does not end here.

Legislation

The second front on which policy initiatives have been taken to insert the federal government in a more robust way into the context of neonatal medical decision making is legislative. The "Child Abuse Amendments of 1984," signed by President Reagan on October 9, 1984, establish a new clause concerned with "Services and Treatment for Disabled Infants." This clause requires state departments of child protection to establish procedures and/or programs to respond to reports of medical neglect, which includes "withholding of medically indicated treatment from disabled infants with life-threatening conditions." "Withholding medically indicated treatment" is defined in the Act as "the failure to respond to the infant's life-threatening conditions by providing treatment (including appropriate nutrition, hydration, and medication) which, in the treating physician's or physicians' reasonable medical judgment, will be most likely to be effective in ameliorating or correcting all such conditions. . . . " Failure to treat for three reasons do not, however, constitute unlawful withholding. These are "when, in the treating physician's or physicians' reasonable medical judgment, (A) the infant is chronically and irreversibly comatose; (B) the provision of such treatment would (i) merely prolong dying, (ii) not be effective in ameliorating or correcting all of the infant's life-threatening conditions, or (iii) otherwise be futile in terms of the survival of the infant; or (C) the provision of such treatment would be virtually futile in terms of the survival of the infant and the treatment itself under such circumstances would be inhumane."[53] Nutrition, hydration, and medication do not fall within the scope of these exceptions. In short, no infant, regardless of condition or prognosis can be denied food, water, or medicine except, presumably, on the basis of "reasonable medical judgment."

The secretary of health and human services is authorized by the amendment to make grants to states for the purpose of fulfilling the requirements of the legislation. Also, grants can be made for informational, educational, or training programs designed to improve professional and paraprofessional services to disabled infants with life-threatening conditions. Parents of disabled infants also qualify as subjects of these programs. Additional funds can be given for program activities that assist in the coordination of services for these infants, including adoption for those qualified. The secretary is required to establish and operate national and regional resource information clearinghouses that will provide the best available information regarding medical treatments and community services for the specified infant population.

As mandated by the amendments, the secretary of HHS issued proposed rules and interim model guidelines for Infant Care Review Committees (ICRC) on December 10, 1984.[54] The proposed rules acknowledge that the protection of children has always been a state and local governmental responsibility. The amendments and proposed rules were intended to extend the scope of this protection to disabled infants[55] with life-threatening conditions. Interventions in these cases have as a primary purpose "to assist parents during this crucial and emotionally difficult time to consider the reasonable medical judgments of their physicians to ensure that proper decisions are made concerning the treatment of these infants."[56] Yet the proposed rules restrict parental choices regarding treatment to the alternatives presented by physicians. Treatment options are determined by "reasonable medical judgment," which is defined to specifically exclude from consideration "subjective 'quality of life' or other abstract concepts."[57]

A bias for treatment, except in those cases specified in the amendments themselves, is underscored by the definition of life-threatening conditions that must be treated. Life-threatening conditions include those that directly threaten life and those that "significantly increase[s] the risk of the onset of complications that may threaten the life of the infant."[58] Thus, open lesions in spina bifida babies and esophageal malformation in Down or Tay-Sachs babies must be treated even though Down syndrome is associated with shortened life and children with Tay-Sachs usually die within five years. Treatment may be legally foregone, according to the proposed rules, if it is "highly unlikely to prevent imminent death" (i.e., "virtually futile") or "the pain and suffering to the infant or other medical contraindications related to 'the treatment itself' clearly outweigh the very slight potential benefit of the treatment for an infant highly unlikely to survive" (i.e., inhumane).[59]

The proposed rules require state agencies to closely cooperate with an ICRC, when available, or a designated hospital-based contact person when conducting an investigation. Hospitals are not required to establish an ICRC, but they are "strongly recommended" to do so. The ICRC is expected to "develop policies and guidelines for the treatment of such infants; act as a resource to hospital personnel and families of disabled infants to provide current and complete information concerning medical treatment, procedures and resources as well as community resources; and review decisions made in individual cases to assure that appropriate treatment is provided. Where medically indicated treatment is not being provided, the ICRC will report such a case to the CPS [Child Protection Services] agency for immediate legal intervention."[60] The ICRC is advised to consult with "medical and other authorities on issues involving treatment and services for disabled individuals"[61] as specific policies and guidelines are drafted. (Curiously, within the list of proposed consultants, parents are not mentioned.) Further, model guidelines are provided for use by an ICRC in the development of its prospective and retrospective review function. The ICRC's activity has as a basic goal, in accord with the amendments and proposed rules, the prevention of withholding medically indicated treatment from impaired infants with life-threatening conditions.[62]

Following a period for public comment, the Department of Health and Human Services issued final rules on April 15, 1985, taking effect one month later.[63] The final rules and the commentary accompanying them constitute an admission that the proposed rules went beyond Congress's intent in amending the Child Abuse Prevention and Treatment Act. In apparent response to objections from the six principal sponsors of the amendment (Senators Hatch, Denton, Cranston, Nickles, Dodd, and Kassebaum) and medical associations, clarifying definitions of "withholding of medically indicated treatment," "life-threatening conditions," "merely prolonging dying," and "virtually futile" were moved from the text to an appendix of the final rule; case examples designed to guide clinicians about the meaning and application of the rule were deleted; and the term "imminent," used in the proposed rule to specify the proximity of death for infants from whom life-prolonging efforts could be withheld, was dropped because its meaning and use would be ambiguous and confusing.[64] Despite these concessions, the department continues to interpret the legislation to exclude "quality of life" considerations from treatment decisions.

A few brief evaluative comments are in order. It should be noted that the federal government is not empowered to become directly involved in individual cases. State agencies are the investigative and enforcement arm of the amendment. Apart from the promise of financial and technical support, the amendment does not seem to confer on state child protection agencies any powers that they did not have. The investigation of allegations of child abuse or neglect is already within their jurisdiction. The amendment appears mainly to encourage an increased concentration of enforcement activity for a class of infants who heretofore were entrusted to the judicious care of parents, physicians, and hospitals until there was cause to think that this trust had been misplaced.

The exceptions to required treatment specified in the amendment and final rules would seem to allow consideration of some quality-of-life criteria in making decisions, despite the department's objections that they do not. For example, life-threatening conditions in irreversibly comatose infants do not require treatment. Presumably, the quality of life of these infants is judged such as to not require support other than food, water, and medicines. If quality-of-life criteria are valid here, why are they as a class excluded from consideration in other cases? Further, it is unclear if medicine in these instances include antibiotics for infections that often kill these patients if left untreated. Presumably, "reasonable medical opinion" can be relied on to make the necessary distinctions in order to act in accord with the law.

Lastly, the exceptions seem to allow for judgments of proportionality regarding the effect of possible treatments. If the negative effects of treatment itself are incommensurate or disproportionate with the "survival," presumably *quality* of survival, it can be considered "inhumane" and not required by the statute. The department's interpretation, however, restricts the criterion of inhumane treatment to cases where it is highly unlikely that the baby will survive even with treatment. A treatment's "inhumaneness" cannot be related, according to the rules, to its effect on the infant's present or future quality of life or impact on the parents. Thus, apart from the stated exceptions it appears, as noted by the AMA,[65] that the department prefers neonatologists and other pediatric specialists to treat correctable defects, without regard for any other handicap an infant may have, no matter how severe or debilitating, except chronic or irreversible coma.

My final comment expresses my major objection to the amended act. It, like its predecessor, the nondiscrimination rules, oversimplifies complex and perplexing moral and medical dilemmas that usually accompany the birth of a severely diseased or anomalous newborn. Though the unique medical circumstances of the infant may be accommodated in the substantive standards of "medically indicated treatment" and "reasonable medical judgment," seemingly neither the particular circumstances of the parents and family, nor their possibly variant but licit moral sense, which may influence a treatment decision, are respected. These rules, like their forerunners, seem to deprive parents, informed by medical and other relevant expertise, of the responsibility and authority to make reasonable treatment decisions for their imperiled infant. In their place, the federal government, after extricating itself ("Baby Doe" squads), has imposed exacting treatment standards (though not always clear) and inserted physicians, a hospital-based informer, and state child protection agencies. Physicians and state child protection agencies were there already. The hospital-based informer is only encouraged. But without the informer, the task of oversight seems not to be changed significantly by the amendments except for an appearance, at least, of distrust of parents and the neonatal team to make reasonable, responsible, and morally defensible treatment decisions for a severely compromised newborn infant. An adversarial atmosphere is fostered where one of compassion, trust, sympathy, patience, understanding, and toleration ought to exist.

Parental Authority Revisited

The desire of policymakers and policy advisors to protect newborn human life, if successful in the manners described above, could have the effect of impairing, on balance, other values, rights, and goods that are, at least, of equal or greater value, in the opinion of this author. The tortuous history of public policy initiatives regarding the medical care of defective newborns has heightened the awareness of professional communities and the public about a profound medical, moral, and legal problem. These policy efforts have generated a new critical reflection on the duties and privileges of parenthood, and the rights and duties of medicine and society vis-à-vis defective infants. It is unfortunate that advocates of a basically full-treatment-regardless-of-defect position tend to view sources of power, specifically the federal government, as a means to coerce or control people's reasonable choices in situations where a single, unqualified right course is nearly always elusive. A moral, more licit use of power, in these ambiguous circumstances, is to respect free, diverse, morally reasonable judgments as a means to secure peace while an inquiry and dialogue ensues.

Regulatory and legislative efforts to impose a disputed, particularly moral judgment regarding who properly decides and the forms of treatment required in cases of reproductive tragedy are thinly veiled grasps at power. In the name of benevolence and disinterest, a particular moral norm is established by the coercive power of government for circumstances where the persuasive force of the supporting reasoning has been found insufficient. A result is that these infants become means to ideological ends. The unique circumstances of each troublesome case militates against supposedly helpful policies based on diagnosis, accompanying handicap, prognosis, bias for full treatment, or bias against any treatment. These ambiguous cases, to use the term employed by the President's Commission, are the main subject of the current controversy. These are the very ones that do not submit very well to preset judgments and standards regarding their care. Indeed, without restrictive policies, particular decisions and actions will appear to some as gross medical and moral mistakes. The same could be said if restrictive policies are set in place. But on balance, it seems that greater harm may come from embarking upon a restrictive course than from pursuing a course that respects freedom and moral diversity, particularly in a society that is characteristically morally pluralistic and secular.

These several policy proposals misperceive the appropriate role of the state in these tragic circumstances. Where reasoned disagreements exist, based on diverse moral visions and derived norms, the state's proper role is that of a neutral observer, acting to protect the freedom of persons to act on their particular, defensible moral judgments. Rather than acting to foreclose or restrict the licit options available to parents, the state, from the moral point of view articulated here, should guard against an unwarranted and unjustified imposition of any single, particular moral vision. This objection to state interference is strengthened by the fact that there is not much evidence to support the claim that the situation of a severely diseased or defective infant for whom treatment is reasonably refused by parents may be improved materially by coercive state intervention.[66]

Placement in institutions is not ideal. A recent study of pediatric nursing homes in Massachusetts found that the residents (most of whom were bedridden, nonverbal, severely or profoundly retarded, and required feeding, dressing, washing, and sensory and motor stimulation) were given less than optimal educational, rehabilitative, and general care.[67] This report suggests that in the case of severely impaired newborns who become institutionalized a preference and respect for reasonable parental judgments may not be ill-advised. And, it should be noted, the potential for harm from state intervention does not fall solely on infants and children.

Labeling parents as unfit, abusive, or neglectful because their reasonable medical-moral judgments do not coincide with others in positions to enforce their view may unjustly stigmatize parents psychologically and socially. Allegations or findings of neglect and abuse may reflect personal values regarding child-rearing rather than clear demonstrations of parental failure. Court proceedings in these cases may be more of a judicial referendum on parental conduct rather than an objective evaluation of the justification for parental conduct and its effect on a child. The understanding of parental autonomy advocated here implies that the state should establish conditions within which parental rights and duties can be acted upon. When a child is healthy the state presumes a congruence of interests between parent and child and a reliability of parental decisions. These same presumptions should exist when a child is ill. As attorney Laurent Frantz reminds us, from the perspective of the law, "it is ordinarily for the parent . . . to decide, . . . what is actually necessary for the protection and preservation of the life and health of his child, so long as he acts as a reasonable and ordinarily prudent parent would act in a like situation."[68]

John Robertson, law professor at the University of Texas, is not convinced that parents of a defective newborn should be free to effectively set aside its right to life by deciding against life-sustaining treatment. He is worried that such a policy leaves the door open for questionable applications to newborns not so seriously impaired, or for otherwise questionable reasons. But, the law recognizes a class of patients for whom prolonged life can be judged reasonably not in their best interest, e.g., Karen Quinlan. Robertson argues that the burden of showing that the state has a compelling interest in a policy that sanctions parental choices for nontreatment of severely impaired newborns has not been met.[69] It seems, however, that Robertson has misplaced the burden of proof. In light of the presumptions of the law regarding parental autonomy, the view of the state endorsed above, and in recognition of the nature of these particular sorts of cases, the burden more accurately appears to rest on those who want to invade the precincts of the family and hospital to impose a norm of conduct that disrespects reasonable judgments and plural moral visions. The Court in *In Re Hofbauer* recognized that reasonable judgments regarding the medical care of children are contextual in nature not easily made subject to hard, fast, and unexceptionable rules.[70]

Those who decide that death for the newborn is, on balance, a grace should realize the seriousness of that decision expressed in the law as homicide and manslaughter.[71] Nevertheless, and in accord with the moral arguments in this volume, if adults have a right to refuse for themselves treatment that is futile or that would result in only a marginal and questionable net benefit, parents should not be restrained, all things considered, from making the same sort of decision for an imperiled newborn whose present and future they hold in trust and for whom they primarily are responsible. Parents, physicians, nurses, and others should be prepared to pay the price that may accompany the exercise of their convictions. The threat of legal retribution can serve as a safeguard against unreasonable and morally indefensible decisions to end newborn human life or to let new life die. Thus I do not advocate now a change in the law. At the same time, I am willing to let the law be ignored when it clearly cannot make a qualitatively better and more defensible decision than parents, or materially improve the net value of life to an imperiled neonate as a result of rescue by forceful state intervention.

Deciding what to do in cases of reproductive tragedy ought to be a private, and not a public, function. Personal, family, religious, and moral issues are involved, and the state is unable to resolve these without the imposition of a vast tyranny,[72] and any form of tyranny is morally objectionable. Its offensiveness is heightened when suffering is compounded and the licit values and commitments of particular moral communities are disrespected. The mutual respect that is basic to a moral pluralism is thereby discarded. Further, the good or least evil that are objects of moral conduct are displaced by other, less morally worthy ends—the imposition by force of a single moral vision. The cases for which a decision for death may be reasonable are those most likely to be the subject of significant disagreement within and between particular moral communities. When this is the case, government ought not impose or seek to impose a decision that respects only one defensible viewpoint. Prosecutors, courts, and legislators properly ought to resist the temptation to dictate a response derived from a single morality where more than one response may have moral sanction. Current homicide and manslaughter statutes are testimony to the high value placed on human life. But in cases where a peaceful and aesthetic death is provided for an infant, judges and juries, if these cases are brought to trial, should be free to accept mercy killing as a defense.

I realize that this stance will be criticized. But in my judgment it is sensible, morally defensible, medically realistic, and legally arguable. It is far better than the alternatives proposed in federal legislation and regulation. In short, I'm prepared to allow parents to choose a reasonably perceived lesser evil for their defective infant rather than endorse the greater evil of unwarranted state intervention that results in a decrease of parental autonomy, authority, and responsibility to exercise the duties of their role. This stance favoring respect for reasonable judgments, in my opinion, is appropriate, given the medical, moral, and legal complexities that are frequently manifested in these cases. Patience and forebearance, in the face of these profound dilemmas, together with a vigilant stand against unreasonable parental choices, are features of a wise and prudent public policy.

CHAPTER

8

Conclusion

Perhaps the only aspect of discussions of moral, medical, policy, and legal quandaries that attend the birth of a severely diseased or defective newborn that is universally agreed upon is that the inquiry and debate will continue. This is as it should be. In a moral environment where diverse visions and senses of moral obligation are acknowledged, controversies of the sort reviewed in this volume, are properly resolved by the persuasive power of reason, not by resort to coercive forms of power. This has been a basic premise behind the expositions and arguments contained in the preceding chapters. The issues and concerns that are characteristic of these tragic circumstances do not admit to a single interpretation, whether the analysis is from a moral, medical, policy, or legal point of view. This is true not only because the factual and theoretical features are subject to varying understandings, but also because of the influence of values that inescapably infuse any consideration of the dilemmas.

Reasons for the unsettled state of affairs with regard to the treatment or nontreatment of defective newborns have been provided in the preceding chapters. It has been shown that neonatology is a context in which the pluralism of the moral community may be displayed. Diverse moral visions, commitments, and norms may be applied to questions of what conduct is morally licit. Controversies may erupt as basic moral and nonmoral values contend for priority. Similarly, the material interests of relevant parties may be brought into conflict. In addition, the negotiation of these controversies and conflicts may result in a choice among relative evils, an end that no one would have preferred, but that everyone may come to accept as the best that could be achieved, all things considered.

The content of parental decisions in situations of reproductive tragedy can be guided by the moral principles of beneficence and justice. The former identifies the good or lesser evil as the proper end of decisions, the latter expands the scope of parental regard to include the relative good and interests of others. The material content of both principles is subject to diverse understandings by particular moral communities and agents within society. There are no widely accepted moral arguments that establish the concrete content of another person's good or due. Differing judgments about what conduct is morally licit in particular circumstances should come as no surprise. To the extent that these diverse judgments are supported by moral arguments, they warrant respect even though other particular moral communities and agents may consider them wrong. Parents of severely diseased or defective newborns may reasonably choose not to authorize life-prolonging interventions when one of several conditions obtain: (1) extended life is reasonably judged not to constitute a net benefit to the infant; (2) it is reasonably believed that the infant's condition is such that the capacities sufficient for a minimal independent existence or personhood in a strict sense cannot be attained; or (3) the costs to other persons, especially parents and family, are sufficient to defeat customary duties of beneficence toward a particular human infant.

Moral support for parental discretion in these matters is further strengthened by an understanding of human neonates as persons in a social sense, rather than as persons in a strict sense. Persons in a strict sense are moral agents, morally self-determining, unqualified members of the moral community, subjects of duties of beneficence, and bearers of rights to forebearance. Newborn human infants, normal or impaired, do not possess the properties or capacities sufficient for unqualified membership in the moral community, are not morally self-determining, or bearers of rights and duties, including those of forebearance and beneficence. Nevertheless, newborn infants can be understood as persons in a social sense because of their role in the moral order. The rights and duties they will bear when they become persons are held in trust for them and exercised in their behalf by parents, in normal circumstances, until a future time and for a future person yet to develop.

This view of parental responsibility and the moral status of newborn humans entails a commensurate understanding of parental authority. This is to say that parents are presumed to be authorities and to have authority to determine the care and nurture of their incompetent children. This authority would encompass judgments regarding the medical care of imperiled newborns that are reasonable under the circumstances and guided by relevant moral principles as interpreted by the particular moral community of which the parents are a part. These decisions warrant respect within a society that acknowledges its pluralism and protects the freedom of particular moral communities and agents to create, discover, and pursue their concrete view of the good. In these situations of reproductive tragedy, parents may conclude, on the basis of their competent understanding of the relevant medical facts, and in accord with their particular moral commitments, that death for an imperiled newborn would be a grace or otherwise morally justified. As the analysis of the alleged moral distinction between killing and letting die showed, a merciful and aesthetic death brought about by direct human intervention is as morally licit in these circumstances as standing by while the mortal process continues unhindered. The role of neonatologists and other members of the neonatal team is that of a sustaining presence, providing competent diagnoses and prognoses based on the best available medical evidence. Understood in this fashion, the neonatal medical team is free to cooperate with parental decisions to the degree that their cooperation does not violate their own moral commitments. Further, public policies that endeavor to override reasonable parental decisions in these matters are unjustified. They misperceive the proper role of the state with regard to parents and this class of infants, and the legal protections appropriate to the moral status of imperiled neonates.

These arguments support a general policy of tolerance of and respect for reasonable parental decisions regarding the treatment, nontreatment, or means of death for that class of severely diseased or defective newborns who satisfy at least one of the several conditions identified above. More specific policies are not morally justified according to the arguments provided here. Neither are they practical. The relevant circumstances of all possible cases are not predictable. Further, it would be difficult to keep them current with the ever-changing capacities of medicine to alter nature's course in these instances.

The defense of parental responsibility and authority with regard to treatment decisions for severely diseased or defective newborns provided here is not intended to disregard or disrespect the value of newborn human life. Neither have I intended to demean or ridicule moral senses and commitments different from those defended in this volume. Rather, the analyses of dilemmas in neonatology provided here are intended to place them in a moral perspective grounded in an understanding of relevant moral principles, informed by relevant research in custom, medicine, and law, and sensitive to the emotional dimensions of these tragic events.

These analyses and conclusions surely are controversial, but, in my judgment, they are defensible and superior to proposals to deprive parents of the responsibility and authority to make reasonable decisions regarding the medical care of their threatened infant. Specific counsel about what to do with very low birth weight, premature, Down syndrome, or spina bifida infants, for example, has not been provided. The burden of decisions in these cases rests properly on responsible parents who are free to make reasonable decisions consistent with their particular moral commitments. Neither has specific direction been given to medical personnel. As a sustaining presence they are enabled to sojourn with parents and newborn down a path often marked by ambivalence, uncertainty, and, perhaps paradoxically, loyalty to the good and the right as it is reasonably discerned by parents in complex and vexing circumstances. In short, the general policy advocated in this volume is one that respects and defends the freedom of present moral agents, regardless of their specific role in situations of reproductive tragedy, to make reasonable decisions and to act in accord with the vision and norms of the particular moral community of which they are a part.

The moral issues and questions related to the medical treatment of imperiled newborn infants will not be settled for everyone by the positions taken in this volume. Further, new dilemmas will emerge as the present limits of neonatal medicine to rescue anomalous newborns are broken. The moral question of whether we ought to do what we can do in every instance of reproductive tragedy will be asked again and again: at times for infants and conditions to which we have become accustomed, (e.g., Down syndrome with operable congenital defects); at other times for treatments that are novel or new (e.g., cross-species transplantation of vital organs). No effort has been made to specify answers for either class of cases. Rather, as I have maintained throughout these pages, the wisdom of particular moral communities and agents are the places to turn for specific guidance. The approach taken here is one in which freedom for moral agents is a value and a constraint upon what may be forced upon present persons without their consent. The moral visions and derived norms of particular communities that generate reasonable choices and conduct in response to complex and perplexing instances of human reproduction warrant respect in a moral pluralism where a single, compelling, concrete view of the good for a particular infant, family, community, and society is lacking. Where moral certainty is missing, where moral judgments are not universally agreed upon, where a moral pluralism is acknowledged and protected, tolerance and respect for considered differences should prevail while an analysis of vexing moral disagreements is sustained. This view holds not only for controversies in neonatology but for every area of moral decision making in which the pluralistic character of the moral community is made manifest by the disagreements that emerge. May we have the wisdom, patience, and courage to perceive the limitations of our particular moral visions and derived norms. And may we have the wisdom, patience, and courage to respect similar limitations that we perceive in the particular moral visions and derived norms of persons with whom we disagree.

Notes

Preface

1. Albert R. Jonsen, Mark Siegler, and William Winslade have authored this sort of volume for use primarily in adult medicine, *Clinical Ethics* (New York: Free Press, 1982).
2. Cf., Robert Weir, *Selective Nontreatment of Handicapped Newborns* (New York: Oxford University Press, 1984), chapters 7–9.

Chapter 1. Introduction

1. John E. Pless, "The Story of Baby Doe," *New England Journal of Medicine* 309 (September 15, 1983): 664.
2. "Notice to Health Care Providers," reported in *The Hastings Center Report* 12 (August 1982): 6.
3. Raymond S. Duff and A. G. M. Campbell, "Moral and Ethical Dilemmas in the Special-Care Nursery," *New England Journal of Medicine* 289 (October 25, 1973): 891.
4. Ted Peters, "Pluralism as a Theological Problem," *The Christian Century* 100 (September 28, 1983): 843.
5. Alasdair MacIntyre, *After Virtue* (Notre Dame, Ind.: University of Notre Dame Press, 1981), p. 6.
6. P. F. Strawson, "Social Morality and Individual Ideal," in *Christian Ethics and Contemporary Philosophy,* edited by I. T. Ramsey (London: SCM Press, 1966), pp. 281–282.

7. For a detailed analysis of the notion of the moral community as it is utilized here, see H. Tristram Engelhardt, Jr., *The Foundations of Bioethics* (New York: Oxford University Press, 1985). According to Engelhardt, the minimum concept of the moral community as a community held together on a basis other than force requires mutual respect by those entities who can conceive of and understand the moral life. Only such entities have moral problems and are objects of unqualified moral respect. The structure of such a broad moral community is found in its procedural agreements, and concrete and relative views of the good life are variously fashioned, discovered, and pursued by particular moral subcommunities and particular moral agents. The life of a particular moral community in a pluralism is justified insofar as it meets the following characteristics: (1) there is mutual respect for the freedom of moral agents; (2) moral controversies are resolved by peaceable means; (3) the free consent of moral agents is the basis of authority; and (4) only persons in a strict sense are unqualified members, persons in a social sense are members because of the roles they have in the community.

8. Tom L. Beauchamp and James F. Childress, *Principles of Biomedical Ethics,* 2nd edition (New York: Oxford University Press, 1983), p. 62.

9. Tom L. Beauchamp and Laurence B. McCullough, *Medical Ethics* (Englewood Cliffs, N.J.: Prentice-Hall, Inc., 1984), pp. 42, 44.

10. Robert M. Veatch, "Limits of Guardian Treatment Refusal: A Reasonableness Standard," *American Journal of Law and Medicine* 9 (Winter 1984): 447. The President's Commission for the Study of Ethical Problems in Medicine and Biomedical Research expresses this idea in the following way: "Especially in a society in which many other traditional forms of community have been eroded, participation in a family is often an important dimension of personal fulfillment. Since a protected sphere of privacy and autonomy is required for the flourishing of this interpersonal union, institutions and the state should be reluctant to intrude, particularly regarding matters that are personal and on which there is a wide range of opinion in society." President's Commission for the Study of Ethical Problems in Medicine and Biomedical and Behavioral Research, *Making Health Care Decisions* (Washington, D.C.: U.S. Government Printing Office, 1982), p. 183.

11. Ibid., p. 442.

12. The adequacy of the standard of reasonableness for decision making on behalf of incompetent patients (e.g., newborns) has been recognized by a presidential Commission that examined the ethical and legal implications of the decision-making process in health care con-

texts. The Commission identified three considerations in making assessments of reasonableness: (1) potential to relieve suffering; (2) probability to preserve or restore functioning; and (3) impact on the value of life to the patient (quality) and the extent life is sustained (p. 180). *Making Health Care Decisions*, pp. 178–180.

13. William L. Prosser, *Law of Torts*, 4th edition (St. Paul, Minn.: West Publishing Co., 1971), pp. 146–150.

14. Ibid., pp. 162–165.

15. Cf., ibid., p. 167.

16. Joseph Goldstein, Anna Freud, and Albert J. Solnit, *Before the Best Interests of the Child* (New York: Free Press, 1979), p. 16.

17. Ibid., p. 91.

18. Cf., Veatch, p. 449.

19. Goldstein, Freud, and Solnit, p. 91. The President's Commission characterized the end to be sought when making decisions for incompetent patients such as newborns as "well-being." Well-being is determined on a case-by-case basis and can include no further intervention, even when health care providers would prefer to intervene. Cf., *Making Health Care Decisions*, pp. 43–44. The Commission's use of well-being seems to roughly correspond to what I mean by "normal healthy growth or a life worth living."

20. Goldstein, Freud, and Solnit, Chapter 5.

21. Goldstein, Freud, and Solnit, pp. 93–94.

22. Ibid.

23. Veatch, p. 433.

24. Ibid., pp. 433–435.

25. See Earl E. Shelp, ed., *Beneficence and Health Care* (Dordrecht, Netherlands: D. Reidel Publishing Co., 1982) for a broad theoretical discussion of the principle of beneficence and its application to health care.

26. Beauchamp and Childress, p. 148. More traditional formulations of the principle of beneficence impose a duty to avoid or lessen evils.

27. Cf., Engelhardt, Chapter 3.

28. Cf., Earl E. Shelp, "To Benefit and Respect Persons: A Challenge for Beneficence in Health Care," in Shelp, pp. 200–217.

29. Cf., John P. Reeder, Jr., "Beneficence, Supererogation, and Role Duty," Natalie Abrams, "Scope of Beneficence in Health Care," and Ronald M. Green, "Altruism in Health Care," in Shelp, *Beneficence and Health Care*, pp. 83–108, 183–198, and 239–254, respectively.

30. Cf., Shelp, "To Benefit and Respect Persons," pp. 204–207.

31. Hans Jonas saw this when he noted that the idea of the primacy of

the individual has achieved axiomatic status in the West. Hans Jonas, "Philosophical Reflections on Experimenting with Human Subjects," in *Ethics in Medicine*, edited by S. J. Reiser, et al. (Cambridge, Mass.: MIT Press, 1977), p. 307.

32. Ibid., p. 305.

33. John Stuart Mill, *On Liberty*, edited by C. V. Shields (Indianapolis, Ind.: Bobbs-Merrill Educational Publishing, 1956), p. 17.

34. Ibid., p. 82.

35. Strawson, pp. 281–282.

36. Ibid., p. 296.

37. For a discussion of theories of justice and their relevance to issues in health care, see Earl E. Shelp, ed., *Justice and Health Care* (Dordrecht, Netherlands: D. Reidel Publishing Co., 1981). See, especially, Albert R. Jonsen, "Justice and the Defective Newborn," pp. 95–107.

38. National Commission for the Protection of Human Subjects of Biomedical and Behavioral Research, *The Belmont Report* (Washington, D.C.: DHEW Publication No. [OS] 78–0012), p. 8.

39. The important issues of macroallocation are being set aside. This is not meant to suggest that the question of what portion of social resources should be dedicated to health care in general and to neonatal care in particular is unimportant. Neither will the microallocational questions of which classes of neonates or which particular neonates should obtain care be discussed. Once again, this level of decision making is of profound moral significance, but the focus of this volume is on decision making by parents for specific neonates. These sidelined issues warrant a more complete scholarly discussion than they have received. Excursuses here would tend to detract from the specific focus of this volume and not add significantly to its conclusions.

40. See Beauchamp and Childress, pp. 187–201, for a general analysis of proposed material principles of justice.

41. The truth of this assertion is demonstrated by the fact of several notions of justice rather than only one (e.g., egalitarian, contractarian, libertarian, utilitarian, and Judeo-Christian). Each reflects a different view of the moral universe, an ideal of the good life, and the means necessary to its approximation. See Allen Buchanan, "Justice: A Philosophical Review," Frederick S. Carney, "Justice and Health Care: A Theological Review," and Earl E. Shelp, "Justice: A Moral Test for Health Care and Health Policy," in Shelp, *Justice and Health Care*, pp. 3–21, 37–50, and 213–229, respectively.

Chapter 2. Parents and Children

1. Plato, *Republic*, V, 457c–d, in *Plato, the Collected Dialogues*, edited by Edith Hamilton and Huntington Cairns (Princeton, N.J.: Princeton University Press, 1961).

2. Ibid., 459d–e, 460c.

3. Plato, *Laws*, VI, 775b–d, in *Plato, the Collected Dialogues*, edited by Edith Hamilton and Huntington Cairns (Princeton, N.J.: Princeton University Press, 1961).

4. Ibid., IX, 869a–c.

5. Aristotle, *Politics*, VII, xvi, translated by Benjamin Jowett (Oxford: Clarendon Press, 1916).

6. Ibid., I. v.; Aristotle *Nicomachean Ethics*, 1160b 20–25, translated by Martin Ostwald (Indianapolis, Ind.: Bobbs-Merrill, 1962).

7. Aristotle, *Politics, II. iii.*

8. Aristotle, *Nicomachean Ethics*, 1159a 30–35.

9. Cicero, *De Officiis*, Chapter 17, translated by Walter Miller (Cambridge, Mass.: Harvard University Press, 1913).

10. Ibid.

11. Ibid., Chapter 18.

12. All scriptural references are to the Revised Standard Version of the Holy Bible. See also *The Jewish Encyclopedia*, s. v. "Family and Family Life," "Marriage"; *The Interpreter's Dictionary of the Bible*, s.v. "Child," "Education, OT.," "Family," "Woman in the OT"; Hans-Ruedi Weber, *Jesus and the Children* (Geneva: World Council of Churches, 1979).

13. The Talmud links the authority of parents to the authority of God (Kiddushin 29a–34a). The nature of this authority and the reverence (fear) and honor owed to the father is indicated in a charming story. "R. Abbahu said, E.g., my son Abimi has fulfilled the precept of honour. Abimi had five ordained sons in his father's lifetime, yet when R. Abbahu came and called out at the door, he himself speedily went and opened it for him, crying, 'yes, yes,' until he reached it. One day he asked him, 'Give me a drink of water.' By the time he brought it he had fallen asleep. Thereupon he bent and stood over him until he awoke" (Kiddushin 31b).

14. St. Augustine, *Of the Morals of the Catholic Church*, Chapter 30, §63, translated by R. Stothert, in *Nicene and Post-Nicene Fathers*, III (Grand Rapids, Mich.: Wm. B. Eerdmans Publishing Co., 1978). In what seems offensive to modern sensitivities, Augustine cites the behavior of the father in the story about Sodom in Genesis 19 as an in-

dication of the extent of parental rights. In the story, a father offers his daughters to an angry group of townsmen rather than violate customs of hospitality and surrender his male houseguests to the mob. Augustine realizes the excesses and abuses that a literal interpretation of this story might occasion. So he cautions, "[I]t is clear that we ought not to take all that we read to have been done by holy or just men, and transfer the same to morals. . . . " Scriptural precedent, according to Augustine, ought not be equated with precept. St. Augustine, *To Consentius: Against Lying*, §20–22, translated by H. Browne, in *The Nicene and Post-Nicene Fathers*, III (Grand Rapids, Mich.: Wm. B. Eerdmans Publishing Co., 1978).

15. St. Augustine, *On the Good of Widowhood*, §18, translated by C. L. Cornish, in *The Nicene and Post-Nicene Fathers*, III (Grand Rapids, Mich.: Wm. B. Eerdmans Publishing Co., 1978).

16. St. Thomas Aquinas, *Summa Theologica*, Q. 41, Art. 1, and Q. 49, Art. 5, translated by the Fathers of the English Dominican Province (London: Burns Oates & Washbourne, Ltd., 1922).

17. Jeffrey Blustein, *Parents and Children* (New York: Oxford University Press, 1982), pp. 56–58.

18. Joseph Gallagher, translator, *The Documents of Vatican II* (New York: Corpus Books, 1966), pp. 249–258.

19. Calvin's thought, remarkably, has been researched very little. Cf., Georgia Harkness, *John Calvin: The Man and His Ethics* (New York: Henry Holt and Company, 1931).

20. John Calvin, *Institutes of the Christian Church* (MacDill AFB, Fla.: MacDonald Publishing Co., n.d.), Book II, Chapter 8, §38; cf., John Calvin, *John Calvin's Sermons on the Ten Commandments*, edited and translated by B. W. Farley (Grand Rapids, Mich.: Baker Book House, 1980).

21. Martin Luther, "The Estate of Marriage, 1522, " in *Luther's Works*, Vol. 45 translated by Walter I. Brandt (Philadelphia: Muhlenberg Press, 1962), p. 46.

22. Ibid., p. 39.

23. Martin Luther, "The Large Catechism," in *The Book of Concord*, edited by Theodore G. Tappert (Philadelphia. Fortress Press, 1959), p. 388.

24. Paul Althaus, *The Ethics of Martin Luther* (Philadelphia: Fortress Press, 1972), pp. 37–38, 99–100.

25. Paul Atlhaus explains Luther's views as reflecting a primitive dualism of good and evil and a mythological concept of the devil. As Augustine cautioned against using the example of the father at Sodom as a precept, Althaus considers Luther's views of the de-

monic insufficient to warrant infanticide of defective newborns. Althaus, pp. 82–83, note 82.

The common secular belief regarding malformed infants was that subhuman creatures stole a normal, healthy human infant and left one of their own in its place. The superstition was that these subhuman creatures envied human beauty and the human immortal soul. Thus, an abnormal infant was not supposed to be human at all, it was subhuman, and not actually borne by the mother. The powers of the underworld were responsible for the misfortune, not the parents. The legends contained instructions regarding certain methods or behaviors believed to protect children from exchange or believed able to reverse the exchange once it had been recognized. The secular belief was strikingly redemptive and compassionate toward the guilt and self-blame that parents of a defective infant might feel. However, the contemporary Christian version of the superstition was not as sensitive. The Christian idea of the changeling identified the devil as the thief of the child. Blame for the misfortune was placed on the parents. These events were allowed, according to the Christian view, because of the sins of the parents. Another version explains that God, being jealous for the parents' love, punishes them for loving their children too much. The most destructive explanation, at least for the mother, was that the birth was the result of sexual intercourse between a woman and the devil. Given the potential severity of social reaction based upon this final explanation, i.e., death of the mother, parents might attempt to keep the birth of a defective infant concealed or to secretly do away with the infant. Cf., Carl Haffter, "The Changeling: History and Psychodynamics of Attitudes to Handicapped Children in European Folklore," *Journal of History of Behavioral Sciences* 4 (1968): 55–61.

Subsequent Protestant theologians who have made more than a passing comment regarding the family, marriage, and parenting have repeated some and revised some of the themes articulated by Luther and Calvin. The divine ordination of marriage, the blessing of children, parental duties to nurture, educate, and spiritually direct children, and the duty of children to honor father and mother are maintained. However, significant revisions of other themes have occurred. The relational goods of marriage have gained emphasis while the procreational purposes have declined. Women are seen as equal with men. Their purpose is no longer seen primarily in terms of their generative capacities. Notions of "responsible parenthood" have gained credibility. In recognition of the increasingly secular nature of social life, the religious ideals for marriage and the family are not seen as normative for people outside of the confessional community on the basis of their theological origin alone. Even within confessional communities, the disparity between the ideal and the actual is acknowledged. Cf., Dietrich Bonhoeffer, *Ethics*, translated by Eberhard Bethge (New York: Macmillan, 1965), and Emil Brunner, *The Divine Imperative* (Philadelphia: Westminster Press, 1947).

26. The material provided here is drawn from several sources: Grace Abbott, *The Child and the State*, Vol. 1 (Chicago: University of Chicago Press, 1938); Philippe Aries, *Centuries of Childhood* (New York: Vintage Books, 1965) and "The Sentimental Revolution," *The Wilson Quarterly* VI (Autumn 1982): 47–53; Aristotle, *Nichomachean Ethics*, translated by Martin Ostwald (Indianapolis, Ind.: Bobbs-Merrill, 1962); William Blackstone, *Commentaries on the Laws of England*, 4 vols. (Chicago: University of Chicago Press, 1979); Blustein, *Parents and Children*; Lloyd deMause, ed., *The History of Childhood* (New York: The Psychohistory Press, 1974); R. H. Feen, "Abortion and Exposure in Ancient Greece," in *Abortion and the Status of the Fetus*, edited by W. B. Bondeson, et al. (Dordrecht, Netherlands: D. Reidel Publishing Co., 1983), pp. 283–300; Barbara Kaye Greenleaf, *Children Through the Ages* (New York: McGraw-Hill, 1978); Edith Hamilton and Huntington Cairns, eds., *Plato: The Collected Dialogues*; Jean-Jacques Rousseau, *Emile* (New York: Basic Books, 1979); Charles E. Rosenberg, ed., *The Family in History* (Philadelphia: University of Pennsylvania Press, 1975); William A. Silverman, "Mismatched Attitudes About Neonatal Death," *Hastings Center Report* 11 (December 1981): 12–16.

27. Philippe Aries repeats the following story from Molière in support of his claim that infants simply did not count in life until their survival seemed probable. "Argan in *Le malade imaginaire* has two daughters, one of marriageable age and little Louison who is just beginning to talk and walk. It is generally known that he is threatening to put his elder daughter in a convent to stop her philandering. His brother asks him: 'How is it, Brother, that rich as you are and having only one daughter, *for I don't count the little one*, you can talk of putting her in a convent?'" Though the story dates from the seventeenth century, its sentiment regarding infants fairly represents the preceding centuries as well. Aries, *Centuries of Childhood*, p. 128.

28. Greenleaf, pp. 48–52.

29. Wet-nursing was justified on several grounds: (1) the weakness of the mother following delivery (maternal mortality also was high); (2) fathers protested against the intrusion between him and his wife that would result from the nursing and other care requirements of the infant; and (3) these tasks were physically and emotionally demanding. Joseph E. Illick, "Child-Rearing in Seventeenth-Century

England and America," in *The History of Childhood*, edited by Lloyd deMause, p. 309.

30. deMause, p. 34.

31. Cited by Illick, p. 326.

32. Blackstone writes, "For the policy of our laws, which are ever watchful to promote industry, did not mean to compel a father to maintain his idle and lazy children in ease and indolence. . . . " Blackstone, Vol. I, p. 437.

33. Ibid., pp. 438–439.

34. Ibid., p. 440.

35. Abbott, p. 193. The laws of Virginia express similar views (Act XXVII, 1646), "whereas sundry laws and statutes by act of parliament established, have with great wisdom ordained, for the better educating of youth in honest and profitable trades and manufactures, as also to avoyd sloath and idlenesse wherewith such young children are easily corrupted, as also for releife of such parents whose poverty extends not to give them breeding, that the justices of the peace should at their discretion, bind out children to tradesmen or husbandmen to be brought up in some good and lawful calling. . . . " pp. 200–201.

36. Thomas Hobbes, *De Corpore Politico*, in *The English Works of Thomas Hobbes*, Vol. 4, edited by William Molesworth (London: John Bohn, 1840), Chapter 4, §3, p. 155.

37. Ibid., §10, pp. 158–159.

38. Thomas Hobbes, *Leviathan: On the Matter, Forme and Power of a Commonwealth Ecclesiastical and Civil*, edited by Michael Oakeshott (New York: Collier Books, 1962), Part II, Chapter 20, pp. 151–158.

39. Blustein, p. 74.

40. John Locke, *Two Treatises of Government*, edited by Thomas I. Cook (New York: Hafner Press, 1947), pp. 7–55.

41. Ibid., pp. 148–149.

42. Ibid., pp. 146–159.

43. Ibid., p. 45.

44. Rousseau writes, "There is no picture more charming than that of the family, but a single missing figure disfigures all the others. If the mother has too little health to be nurse, the father will have too much business to be preceptor. The children, sent away, disposed in boarding schools, convents, colleges, will take the love belonging to the paternal home elsewhere, or to put it better, they will bring back to the paternal home the habit of having no attachments. Brothers and sisters will hardly know one another. When all are gathered together for ceremonial occasions, they will be able to be

quite polite with one another. They will treat one another as strangers. As soon as the society of the family no longer constitutes the sweetness of life, it is of course necessary to turn to bad morals to find a substitute." Jean-Jacques Rousseau, *Emile: or On Education*, translated by Allan Bloom (New York: Basic Books, 1979), p. 49.

45. Jeremy Bentham, *The Theory of Legislation* (New York: Harcourt, Brace and Co., 1931), p. 211.

46. Henry Sidgwick, *The Methods of Ethics*, 7th edition (Indianapolis, Ind.: Hackett Publishing Co., 1981), p. 249.

47. Ibid., p. 248, note 1.

48. Cf., Alexander Morgan Capron, "The Authority of Others to Decide About Biomedical Interventions with Incompetents," in *Who Speaks for the Child: The Problems of Proxy Consent*, edited by Willard Gaylin and Ruth Macklin (New York: Plenum Press, 1982), p. 117.

49. 59 Am Jur 2d, Parent and Child, p. 90.

50. Joseph Goldstein, "Medical Care for the Child at Risk: On State Supervention of Parental Autonomy," in Gaylin and Macklin, p. 154.

51. *Griswold* v. *Connecticut*, 381 U.S. 479, 485–86 (1965).

52. *Educ.* v. *LaFleur*, 414, U.S. 632, 639–640 (1970); *Roe* v. *Wade, 410 U.S. 113, 152–153 (1972)*; *Meyer* v *Nebraska*, 262 U.S. 390, 400–403 (1923).

53. *Pierce* v. *Society of Sisters*, 268 U.S. 510, 534–534 (1925).

54. *Wisconsin* v. *Yoder*, 406 U.S. 205, 230–235 (1972).

55. Elizabeth S. MacMillan, "Birth-Defective Infants: A Standard for Nontreatment," *Stanford Law Review* 30 (February 1978): 610.

56. Stuart J. Baskin, "State Intervention into Family Affairs: Justifications and Limitations," *Stanford Law Review* 26 (June 1974): 1383–1409.

57. Joseph Goldstein, Anna Freud, and Albert J. Solnit, *Beyond the Best Interests of the Child* (New York: Free Press, 1973), p. 3. These authors discuss the grounds for state intervention with parental decisions regarding medical care for children in *Before the Best Interests of the Child* (New York: Free Press, 1979), pp. 91–109.

58. Ibid., p. 9.

59. *In Re Hofbauer*, 419 N.Y. 2d 940.

60. Goldstein, Freud, and Solnit, *Beyond the Best Interests of the Child*, pp. 49–50.

61. 59 Am Jur 2d, Parent and Child, p. 138.

62. Laurence H. Tribe, "The Supreme Court, 1972 Term—Forward: Toward a Model of Roles in the Due Process of Life and Law," *Harvard Law Review* 87 (1973): 35–36.

63. 59 Am Jur 2d, Parent and Child, pp. 144–145.

64. MacMillan, p. 610.

65. "Developments in the Law: The Constitution and the Family," *Harvard Law Review* 93 (April 1980): 1198–1199.

66. Michael Wald, "State Intervention on Behalf of 'Neglected' Children: A Search for Realistic Standards," *Stanford Law Review* 27 (April 1975): 1001.

67. Baskin, pp. 1386–1387.

68. Capron, pp. 144, 151–152.

69. *Parham* v. *J. R.*, 422 U.S. 584, 602.

70. Ibid., pp. 602–603.

71. These capacities, even when minimally present, seem to reflect those activities and abilities usually associated with normal human existence. They are valued because, at least in part, their joint presence enables life to be of use to the one who lives it and to others. I fully expect and welcome a sustained discussion of the validity of the standard of independence and its criteria. The proposals made here indicate what I presently think about this matter. These thoughts are tentative in that I am open to data and arguments that displace the normativeness of the goal or the validity of the criteria with regard to newborns. I am *not* proposing the standard or criteria should be applied to beings who once were independent but are not now or ever will be again. Clearly the standard and criteria have implications regarding our duties toward these individuals but these matters are explicitly set aside here.

Chapter 3. Critically Ill Newborns: Parental Responses and Responsibilities

1. Sar A. Levitan and Richard S. Belous, *What's Happening to the American Family?* (Baltimore, Md.: Johns Hopkins University Press, 1981), p. 41.

2. U.S. Department of Commerce, Bureau of the Census, *Statistical Abstract of the United States, 1982–83* (Washington, D.C.: U.S. Government Printing Office, 1982), p. 68.

3. Ibid.; Melinda Beck and Diane Weathers, "America's Abortion Dilemma," *Newsweek* 104 (January 14, 1985): 20.

4. Bureau of the Census, *Statistical Abstract 1982–83*, pp. 60–61.

5. U.S. Department of Commerce, Bureau of the Census, *Statistical Abstract of the United States, 1984* (Washington, D.C.: U.S. Government Printing Office, 1984), p. 47.

6. Ibid., p. 53.

7. Levitan and Belous, pp. 52–54, 59.

8. Bureau of the Census, *Statistical Abstract, 1982–83*, p. 67.

9. Jeffrey Blustein, *Parents and Children* (New York: Oxford University Press, 1982), pp. 148–149.

10. Cf., Albert J. Solnit and Mary H. Stark, "Mourning and the Birth of a Defective Child," *Psychoanalytic Study of the Child* 16 (1961): 523–537.

11. John D. Biggers, "In Vitro Fertilization, Embryo Culture and Embryo Transfer in the Human," in *Appendix: HEW Support of Research Involving Human In Vitro Fertilization and Embryo Transfer*, Ethics Advisory Board, Department of HEW, May 4,1979 (Washington, D.C.), #8, pp. 7, 11. See also John D. Biggers, "Generation of the Human Life Cycle," in *Abortion and the Status of the Fetus*, edited by W. B. Bondeson, et al. (Dordrecht, Netherlands: D. Reidel Publishing Co., 1983), pp. 31–53.

12. *New York Times*, January 22, 1984, p. E5.

13. Barbara R. Grumet, "Reproductive Freedom and the Prevention of Birth Defects: A New and Developing Standard of Medical Care," *Medicolegal News* 8 (October 1980): 5.

14. Daniel Bergsma, ed., *Birth Defects Compendium*, 2nd edition (New York: The National Foundation, March of Dimes, 1979).

15. Walter S. Feldman, "Passive Euthanasia Revisited," *Legal Aspects of Medical Practice*, March 1983, p. 6.

16. Bureau of the Census, *Statistical Abstract, 1982–83*, p. 63.

17. President's Commission for the Study of Ethical Problems in Medicine and Biomedical and Behavioral Research, *Deciding to Forego Life-Sustaining Treatment* (Washington, D.C.: U.S. Government Printing Office, 1983), p. 201.

18. Feldman, p. 6.

19. For a discussion of the transition to parenthood, see Lois Wandersman, Abraham Wandersman, and Steven Kahn, "Social Support in the Transition to Parenthood," *Journal of Community Psychology* 8 (1980): 332–342.

20. Pauline C. Cohen, "The Impact of the Handicapped Child on the Family," *Social Casework* 43 (1962): 137–142.

21. Peggy Muller Miezio, *Parenting Children with Disabilities* (New York: Marcel Dekker, Inc., 1983), p. 10.

22. Robert Stinson and Peggy Stinson, *The Long Dying of Baby Andrew* (Boston: Little Brown and Company, 1983), p. 39.

23. Ibid., pp. 52 and 239.

24. Cf., Rosalyn B. Darling and Jon Darling, *Children Who Are Different: Meeting the Challenge of Birth Defects in Society* (St. Louis, Mo.: C. V. Mosby Co., 1982), pp. 31 and 36.

25. Ethel Roskies, *Abnormality and Normality: The Mothering of Thalidomide Children* (Ithaca, N.Y.: Cornell University Press, 1972), pp. 278 and 283.

26. Murdina M. Desmond, Abbie L. Vorderman, and Martha Salinas, "The Family and Premature Infant After Neonatal Intensive Care," *Texas Medicine* (reprint, no date).

27. Miezio, pp. 10–11.

28. M. M. Desmond, et al., "The Very Low Birth-Weight Infant After Discharge From Intensive Care: Anticipatory Health Care and Developmental Course," *Current Problems in Pediatrics* 10 (April 1980): 13.

29. Cf., N. A. Irvin, J. H. Kennell and M. H. Klaus, "Caring for the Parents of an Infant with a Congenital Malformation," in *Parent-Infant Bonding*, 2nd edition, edited by M. H. Klaus and J. H. Kennell (St. Louis, Mo.: C. V. Mosby Co., 1982), pp. 233–237.

30. James M. Gustafson, "Mongolism, Parental Desires, and the Right to Life," *Perspectives in Biology and Medicine* 16 (Summer 1973): 529–557.

31. For a discussion of the ordinary and extraordinary distinction within Roman Catholic moral theology see Gerald Kelly, *Medico-Moral Problems* (St. Louis, Mo.: Catholic Hospital Association, 1958). This distinction also is employed by non-Catholics: Tom L. Beauchamp and James F. Childress, *Principles of Biomedical Ethics*, 2nd edition (New York: Oxford University Press, 1983), pp. 126–136, and President's Commission, *Deciding to Forego Life-Sustaining Treatment* Chapter 2, esp. pp. 82–89.

32. 76 Am Jur 2d, Trust, §326.

33. 29 Am Jur 2d, Guardian and Ward, §6.

34. An interpretation of Hegel's view of the nation-state may be helpful in appreciating the autonomy with which parents, as quasi-trustees of their children, should be free to perform their duties. Hegel thought of the nation-state as that which transcends particular civil societies and facilitates the pursuit of each society's respective goods. In other words, the nation-state provides a neutral matrix within which particular communities express themselves. This form of service by the nation-state is vitally important in societies in which a common view of the good life is not shared. Within a pluralism, many particular communities with individual and differing visions of the good life exist beside one another; they may also compete in peaceable ways for adherents. The nation-state, according to this interpretation of Hegel, does not take sides or seek to establish one vision of the good life, and its derivative moral norms, to the exclusion of other visions and derived norms. Rather, the state exists to

facilitate within its jurisdiction the freedom of individuals and particular communities to pursue their respective good. In short, the state should be a neutral observer and facilitator for parents to properly perform their duties as parents (quasi-trustees) of dependent children. Cf., T. M. Knox, trans., *Hegel's Philosophy of Right* (London: Oxford University Press, 1967). H. Tristram Engelhardt, Jr., has helped me to understand Hegel's views.

Chapter 4. Neonatal Medicine:
A Context of Intersecting Interests

1. Owsei Temkin, trans., *Soranus' Gynecology* (Baltimore, Md.: Johns Hopkins University Press, 1956), pp. 79–80.

2. Harry H. Gordon, "Perspectives on Neonatology—1980," in *Ethics of Newborn Intensive Care,* edited by Albert R. Jonsen and Michael J. Garland (Berkeley, Calif.: Health Policy Program and Institute of Government Studies, University of California, 1976), p. 3; and William A. Silverman, "Incubator-Baby Side Shows," *Pediatrics* 64 (August 1979): 128–129. Budin's observations are confirmed by contemporary pediatricians. Sibylle K. Escalona reports that small for gestational age and premature infants are more vulnerable to environmental inadequacies posthospitalization than term babies. They also are found to have higher rates of major and minor neurologic and developmental abnormalities than term babies. See Sibylle K. Escalona, "Babies at Double Hazard: Early Development of Infants at Biologic and Social Risk," *Pediatrics* 70 (November 1982): 670–676. See also Betty R. Vohr and William Oh, "Growth and Development in Preterm Infants Small for Gestational Age," *Journal of Pediatrics* 103 (December 1983):941–945; J. O. O. Commey and P. M. Fitzhardinge, "Handicap in the Preterm Small-for-Gestational Age Infant," *Journal of Pediatrics* 94 (May 1979): 799–786; Saroj Saigal, et al., "Follow-up of Infants 501 to 1,500 gm Birth Weight Delivered to Residents of a Geographically Defined Region with Perinatal Intensive Care Facilities," *Journal of Pediatrics* 100 (April 1982): 606–613; John M. Driscoll, et al., "Mortality and Morbidity in Infants Less Than 1,001 Grams Birth Weight," *Pediatrics* 69 (January 1982): 21–26; Maria P. D. Ruiz, et al., "Early Development of Infants of Birth Weight Less than 1,000 Grams with Reference to Mechanical Ventilation in Newborn Period," *Pediatrics* 68 (September 1981): 330–334.

3. Cited by Silverman, p. 129. There is much in this article of value with regard to Couney and the development of incubators.

4. Ibid., p. 140.

5. Gordon, pp. 4 and 8, It is still true that at-risk babies are at de-creased risk of mortality and morbidity when born at a hospital with neonatal intensive care thus reducing the risk associated with trans-port. Cf., J. O. O. Commey and P. M. Fitzhardinge, "Handicap in the Preterm Small-for-Gestational Age Infant"; S. Bennett Britton, P. M. Fitzhardinge, and S. Ashby, "Is Intensive Care Justified for Infants Weighing Less Than 801 gm at Birth?" *Journal of Pediatrics* 99 (December 1981): 937–943; Savitri P. Kumar, et al., "Follow-up Stud-ies of Very Low Birth Weight Infants (1,250 Grams or Less) Born and Treated Within a Perinatal Center," *Pediatrics* 66 (September 1980): 438–444.

6. Clement A. Smith, "Neonatal Medicine and Quality of Life: An His-torical Perspective," in Jonsen and Garland, p. 33.

7. Peter Budetti, et al., *The Implications of Cost-Effectiveness Analysis of Medical Technology: Case Study #10; The Costs and Effectiveness of Neo-natal Intensive Care* (Washington, D.C.: U.S. Government Printing Office, 1980), p. 8.

8. Cf., Stanley N. Graven, "The Organization of Perinatal Health Ser-vices," in *Neonatal-Perinatal Medicine*, 2nd. edition, edited by Rich-ard E. Behrman (St. Louis, Mo.: C. V. Mosby Co., 1977), pp. 7–8; and Paul R. Swyer, "The Organization of Perinatal Care with Par-ticular Reference to the Newborn," in *Neonatology*, 2nd. edition, ed-ited by Gordon B. Avery (Philadelphia: J. B. Lippincott Co., 1981), p. 18.

9. Table reproduced from Graven, p. 8, and other information from Graven, pp. 6–8, and Swyer, p. 33.

10. Ibid., p. 6. See, for example, Jonsen and Garland.

11. Swyer, p. 17.

12. Peter P. Budetti and Peggy McManus, "Assessing the Effectiveness of Neonatal Intensive Care," *Medical Care* 20 (October 1982): 1027. Cf., N. Paneth, et al., "Newborn Intensive Care and Neonatal Mor-tality in Low-Birth-Weight Infants," *New England Journal of Medicine* 307 (July 15, 1982): 149–155. This report based on experiences in New York City suggests that Level 3 care does reduce mortality in low birth weight infants.

13. Budetti, et al., p. 5. Note that Budetti says "probably declining." There is a significant debate about declining morbidity, especially for preterm and low birth weight infants.

14. From the twentieth week of gestation through twenty-eight days following birth.

15. Kwang-Sun Lee, et al., "Neonatal Mortality: An Analysis of the Re-cent Improvement in the United States," *American Journal of Public Health* 70 (1980): 15.

16. Infant mortality is death under one year of age.

17. Budetti and McManus, p. 1029.

18. Jack Hadley, *More Medical Care, Better Health?* (Washington, D.C.: Urban Institute Press, 1982), pp. 33–34.

19. Budetti and McManus, p. 1031. Similarly, since the introduction of ventilatory support for premature infants, prospects for survival have increased, particularly after twenty-eight weeks of gestation.

SURVIVAL BY WEEK OF GESTATION

Weeks	1970–71	1975–76
26	< 10%	> 20%
28	< 30%	< 70%
30	> 80%	> 90%
32	< 90%	> 90%
34	< 90%	> 90%

(< = less than; > = greater than)

M. M. Desmond, et al., "The Very Low Birth Weight Infant After Discharge From Intensive Care: Anticipatory Health Care and Developmental Course," *Current Problems in Pediatrics* 10 (April 1980): 6.

20. Critical reports: Ruiz, et al., "Early Development of Infants of Birth Weight Less Than 1,000 Grams with Reference to Mechanical Ventilation"; Alan D. Rothberg, et al., "Infants Weighing 1,000 Grams or Less at Birth: Developmental Outcome for Ventilated and Non-ventilated Infants," *Pediatrics* 71 (April 1983): 599–602. Optimistic reports: R. S. Cohen, et al., "Favorable Results of Neonatal Intensive Care for Very Low-Birth-Weight Infants," *Pediatrics* 69 (May 1982): 621–625; Alan D. Rothberg, et al., "Outcome for Survivors of Mechanical Ventilation Weighing Less Than 1,250 gm. at Birth," *Journal of Pediatrics* 98 (January 1981): 106–111.

21. Budetti, et al., p. 33. Serious handicap was understood as severe mental retardation (I.Q. less than 70), neurologic defect, particularly cerebral palsy of significant degree, major seizure disorders, and retrolental fibroplasia with blindness or significant visual impairment.

22. Ibid., p. 37. The OTA report observes that prior to 1960 approximately 24 percent of survivors weighing 52 1/2 ounces (1,500 grams) or less had serious handicaps. After 1965 the number dropped to 13.6 percent. The smaller infants weighing 35 ounces (1,000 grams) or less seem also to have fared better. Prior to 1965, approximately 29 percent survived with serious handicap. After 1965, the percentage has been cut almost in half to 16 percent.

23. Ibid., pp. 34–35.

24. Cf., S. P. Horwood, et al., "Mortality and Morbidity of 500-to-1,499-

Gram Birth Weight Infants Live-born to Residents of a Defined Geographic Region Before and After Neonatal Intensive Care," *Pediatrics* 69 (May 1982): 617–618; and Britton, Fitzhardinge, and Ashby, "Is Intensive Care Justified for Infants Weighing Less Than 801 gm. at Birth?" See also studies in the United States: Driscoll, et al., "Mortality and Morbidity in Infants Less Than 1,001 Grams Birth Weight"; Vohr and Oh, "Growth and Development in Preterm Infants Small for Gestational Age"; and Forrest C. Bennett, Nancy M. Robinson, and Clifford J. Sells, "Growth and Development of Infants Weighing Less Than 800 Grams at Birth," *Pediatrics* 71 (March 1983): 319–323. Studies in Canada: Commey and Fitzhardinge, "Handicap in the Preterm Small-for-Gestational Age Infant"; Saigal, et al., "Follow-up of Infants 501 to 1,500 gm. Birth Weight Delivered to Residents of a Geographically Defined Region with Perinatal Intensive Care Facilities." Two additional reports warrant attention: Rosamond A. K. Jones, Mary Cummins, and Pamela A. Davis, "Infants of Very Low Birthweight: A 15-year Analysis," *Lancet* (June 23, 1979): 1332–1335; and S. Shapiro, et al., "Relevance of Correlates of Infant Deaths for Significant Morbidity at 1 Year of Age," *American Journal of Obstetrics & Gynecology* 136 (February 1, 1980): 364 and 369.

25. J. J. Pomerance, et al., "Cost of Living for Infants Weighing 1,000 Grams or Less at Birth," *Pediatrics* 61 (June 1978): 908–910. Pomerance reported the hospital charges for the care of seventy-five high-risk infants weighing 35 ounces (1,000 grams) or less. Thirty survived and 19 out of 27 tested (70 percent) appeared neurologically and developmentally "normal" at one to three years of age. Adjusted to September 1976 rates and excluding charges for physicians' services, the average daily cost per nonsurvivor was $825, with an average total cost of $14,236. For the thirty survivors, the average daily cost was $450, with an average total cost of $40,287. Total costs for all infants were adjusted to determine the average total cost per "normal" survivor ($88,058). The total adjusted cost for the thirty survivors was $1,208,582, for survivors and nonsurvivors it was $1,849,216 stated in 1976 dollars.

A more recent study by C. S. Phibbs and colleagues found upon analysis of 1,185 admissions to the intensive care nursery at H. C. Moffett Hospital in San Francisco that cost variations are related to three risk factors: low birth weight, surgical intervention, and assisted ventilation. Infants weighing 52 1/2 ounces (1,500 grams) or less represented 18 percent of all cases but incurred 37 percent of all costs. Infants requiring surgery constituted 18 percent of admissions but generated 43 percent of total costs. And the costs of producing a survivor who required assisted ventilation was more than

4 1/2 times that of unassisted survivors. See C. S. Phibbs, R. L. Williams, and R. H. Phibbs, "Newborn Risk Factors and Costs of Neonatal Intensive Care," *Pediatrics* 68 (September 1981): 313–321.

26. Michael H. Boyle, et al., "Economic Evaluation of Neonatal Intensive Care of Very-Low-Birth-Weight Infants," *New England Journal of Medicine* 308 (June 2, 1983): 1335.

27. See, for example, Raymond S. Duff and A. G. M. Campbell, "Moral and Ethical Dilemmas in the Special-Care Nursery," *New England Journal of Medicine* 289 (October 25, 1973): 890–894; John Lorber, "Results of Treatment of Myelomeningocele," *Developmental Medicine and Child Neurology* 13 (1971): 279–303; and John Lorber, "Early Results of Selective Treatment of Spina Bifida Cystica," *British Medical Journal* 4 (1973): 201–204.

28. Cf., Robert M. Veatch, "Models for Ethical Medicine in a Revolutionary Age: What Physician-Patient Roles Foster the Most Ethical Relationship," *Hastings Center Report* 2 (June 1972): 5–7; Robert M. Veatch, *A Theory of Medical Ethics* (New York: Basic Books, 1981); William F. May, "Code and Covenant or Philanthropy and Contract," in *Ethics in Medicine,* edited by Stanley J. Reiser, Arthur J. Dyck, and William J. Curran, (Cambridge, Mass.: MIT Press, 1977), pp. 65–76; May, *The Physician's Covenant* (Philadelphia: Westminster Press, 1983); Roger D. Masters, "Is Contract an Adequate Basis for Medical Ethics," *Hastings Center Report* 5 (December 1975): 24–28.

29. Models or images of physicians perform three functions: they define a social role; they reveal a perception of the condition of human existence; and they serve as a guide to practice. May, *The Physician's Covenant,* pp. 16–20.

30. Ibid., pp. 23–24.

31. Veatch (contract) considers himself and May (covenant) to be in essential agreement. Cf., Robert M. Veatch, "The Case of Contract in Medical Ethics," in *The Clinical Encounter,* edited by Earl E. Shelp (Dordrecht, Netherlands: D. Reidel Publishing Co., 1983), pp. 105–112.

32. Different versions of the discussion that follows appeared in Earl E. Shelp, "Courage: A Neglected Virtue in the Patient-Physician Relationship," *Social Science & Medicine* 18, (1984): 351–360, and in Earl E. Shelp, "Courage and Tragedy in Clinical Medicine," *Journal of Medicine and Philosophy* 8 (November 1983): 417–429.

33. A cure–least evil pattern for the range of legitimate ends of the patient-physician relationship is suggestive but too simplistic. Anything more specific, however, would risk excluding valid ends within these parameters.

34. Cf., Eric J. Cassell, *The Healer's Art* (Philadelphia: J. B. Lippincott, 1976), p. 182.

35. Cf., Eric J. Cassell, "The Nature of Suffering and the Goals of Medicine," *New England Journal of Medicine* 306 (1982): 639–645.

36. Cf., Stanley Hauerwas, "Medicine as a Tragic Profession," in *Truthfulness and Tragedy*, by Stanley Hauerwas with R. Bondi and D. B. Burrell (Notre Dame, Ind.: University of Notre Dame Press, 1977), pp. 184–202.

37. Cf., Robert Weir, *Selective Nontreatment of Handicapped Newborns* (New York: Oxford University Press, 1984), pp. 257–271.

38. Ibid., p. 262.

39. Ibid.

40. Ibid.

41. Ibid., p. 197.

42. Ibid., p. 198.

43. Ibid., p. 268.

44. James F. Childress, *Who Should Decide?* (New York: Oxford University Press, 1982), pp. 172–174.

45. Weir, p. 269.

46. Ibid.

47. Whether informed consent ever takes place is debated. It is not necessary to settle this question here. All that requires notice is that comprehension and competency are criteria for informed treatment decisions, regardless of who the decider is.

48. I and a psychiatric colleague have discussed these matters in slightly different form in "Denial in Clinical Medicine," *Archives of Internal Medicine* 145 (April 1985): 697–699; and H. T. Engelhardt, Jr., M. A. Gardell, and E. E. Shelp, eds. *Competent Patients as Incompetents* (Dordrecht, Netherlands: D. Reidel Publishing Co., forthcoming).

49. The Judicial Council of the American Medical Association recently concurred that "the decision whether to exert maximal efforts to sustain life should be the choice of parents. . . . The presumption is that the love which parents usually have for their children will be dominant in the decisions which they make in determining what is in the best interest of their children." Judicial Council of the American Medical Association, *Current Opinions, 1982* (Chicago: American Medical Association, 1982), p. 9.

50. Weir, pp. 258–259.

51. Ibid, pp. 259–260.

52. Ibid, p. 260.

Chapter 5. Making Treatment Decisions

1. Cf., V. Apgar and L. S. James, "Further Observations on the New-born Scoring System," *American Journal of Diseases of Children* 104 (October 1962): 419–428.

2. Robert S. Morison, "Is There a Biological Person?" *Milbank Memorial Fund Quarterly/Health and Society* 61 (Winter 1983): 17.

3. Cf., Daniel Callahan, *Abortion: Law, Choice and Morality* (New York: Macmillan 1970), pp. 355ff.

4. Charles Hartshorne, "Scientific and Religious Aspects of Bioethics," in *Theology and Bioethics*, edited by Earl E. Shelp (Dordrecht, Netherlands: D. Reidel Publishing Co., 1985), p. 34.

5. Ruth Macklin, "Personhood in the Bioethics Literature," *Milbank Memorial Fund Quarterly/Health and Society* 61 (Winter 1983): 52.

6. John T. Noonan, Jr., "From 'An Almost Absolute Value in History,'" in *Moral Problems in Medicine*, edited by Samuel Gorovitz, et al. (Englewood Cliffs, N.J.: Prentice Hall, 1976), pp. 294–296, *inter alia*.

7. Cf., Albert S. Moraczewski, "Human Personhood: A Study in Personalized Biology," in *Abortion and the Status of the Fetus*, edited by William B. Bondeson, H. T. Engelhardt, Jr., S. F. Spicker, and D. H. Winship (Dordrecht, Netherlands: D. Reidel Publishing Co., 1983), p. 309.

8. Leonard J. Weber, *Who Shall Live?* (New York: Paulist Press, 1976), p. 42.

9. Morison, pp. 8–9, 15.

10. Cf., S. Bok, "Death and Dying: Euthanasia and Sustaining Life: II. Ethical Views," *Encyclopedia of Bioethics* (New York: Macmillan–Free Press, 1978), pp. 272–274; R. A. McCormick, "Ambiguity in Moral Choice," in *Doing Evil to Achieve Good*, edited by R. A. McCormick and P. Ramsey (Chicago: Loyola University Press, 1978), pp. 7–53; and P. Foot, "The Problem of Abortion and the Doctrine of Double Effect," in *Virtue and Vice* (Berkeley: University of California Press, 1978), pp. 19–32.

11. A. G. M. van Melsen, "Person," *Encyclopedia of Bioethics*, p. 1207.

12. Joseph F. Fletcher, "Four Indicators of Humanhood—The Enquiry Matures," *Hastings Center Report* 4 (December 1974): 4–7.

13. Mary Anne Warren, "On the Moral and Legal Status of Abortion," in *Contemporary Issues in Bioethics*, edited by Tom L. Beauchamp and LeRoy Walters, (Belmont, Calif.: Dickenson Publishing Co., 1978), p. 224.

14. Singer explains his preference for self-consciousness in the follow-

ing way: "As long as a sentient being is conscious, it has an interest in experiencing as much pleasure and as little pain as possible. Sentience suffices to place a being within the sphere of equal consideration of interests: but it does not mean that the being has a personal interest in continuing to live. For a non-self-conscious being, death is the cessation of experiences, in much the same way that birth is the beginning of experiences. Death cannot be contrary to an interest in continued life, any more than birth could be in accordance with an interest in commencing life. To this extent, with non-self-conscious life, birth and death cancel each other out; whereas with self-conscious beings the fact that once self-conscious one may desire to continue living means that death inflicts a loss for which the birth of another is insufficient compensation," Peter Singer, *Practical Ethics* (Cambridge, Mass.: Cambridge University Press, 1979), pp. 102–103.

15 Michael Tooley, *Abortion and Infanticide* (New York: Oxford University Press, 1983), p. 134. The content of this person-making property is as follows: (1) The desires in question must either be (at least potentially) represented in consciousness, or be directed at states of consciousness. (2) The interrelationships among these desires must satisfy the following: (a) they must be desires had by the same mental substance or subject of consciousness; (b) there must be psychological continuity among the desires; (c) the desires must be linked together by memory beliefs concerning the existence of earlier desires associated with the same mental substance; (d) earlier desires must be accompanied by beliefs that there will be later desires belonging to the same mental substance; (e) earlier desires must be accompanied by desires for the existence of later desires belonging to the same mental substance.

Tooley refrains from asserting that this property is also necessary for personhood, but it is clear that he thinks it probably is. Other candidates for person-making characteristics that have traditionally been given—species membership, rationality, capacity for intentional action, self-consciousness—are either rejected or accepted only insofar as they are in some way related to the concept of having nonmomentary interests. Being the subject of nonmomentary interests entails necessarily for Tooley that the entity having beliefs/desires possess a concept of a continuing self, i.e., of a substance that will continue through time and, thus, be *the same* substance existing at some later time. Only those substances or entities subject to nonmomentary interests or possessing the concept of a continuing self have a right to continued existence.

Tooley attempts to link being a subject of rights with being capable of having interests and desires. He asks, "What must be the

case if the continued existence of something is to be in its interest?''
(p. 118). An answer is derived from a consideration of two hypo-
thetical cases. Case one: A human embryo that has not yet developed to the point at which it would be capable of having any desires,
or indeed any conscious states at all, but which will develop into a
happy individual who will be glad that it was not aborted. Is it in
the interest of this embryo that it continue to exist? Tooley considers
the following possible justification for an affirmative answer. Suppose Mary is the individual who results from the development of
the embryo into a happy person. Surely it was in Mary's interest
that a certain embryo was not destroyed once upon a time. But Mary
is the same individual as the embryo in question. Therefore, it was
in the embryo's interest not to be destroyed, i.e., to continue to
exist. Tooley's attack on this line of reasoning appeals to his contention that a subject of interests must be a subject of conscious
states, particularly desires. "This means that in identifying Mary
with the embryo, and attributing to it her interest in its earlier non-
destruction, one is treating the embryo as if it were itself a subject
of consciousness'' (p. 119). But by hypothesis the embryo is not a
subject of consciousness. Thus, it cannot have any interests at all;
in particular, it cannot have an interest in its continued existence.

Case two: A human baby that has developed to the point of having simple desires but does not yet have the capacity for desiring
its own continued existence. The baby will have a happy life, and
will be glad it was not destroyed. Does this baby have a right to
continued existence? Tooley considers the following affirmative response: "If Mary is the resulting individual, then it was in Mary's
interest that the baby not have been destroyed. But the baby just *is*
Mary when she was young. So it must have been in the baby's interest that it not have been destroyed'' (p. 119). Tooley's response
in this case must be different from that in case one because the baby
in question here *is* a subject of consciousness and of desires. He is
willing to allow that if there is psychological continuity between the
baby and the later Mary, then the conclusion that it was in the baby's interest not to be destroyed is valid. Tooley continues, "On the
other hand, suppose that not only does Mary, at a much later time,
not remember any of the baby's experiences, but the experiences in
question are not psychologically linked, either by memory or in any
other way, to mental states enjoyed by the human organism in question at *any* later time. Here it seems to me clearly incorrect to say
that Mary and the baby are one and the same subject of consciousness, and therefore it cannot be correct to transfer, from Mary to the
baby, Mary's interest in the baby's not having been destroyed'' (p.
119–120). The operative principle in this criticism seems to be the

following: If it is in A's interest at some time t_2 that p, then it was in A's interest at some earlier time t_1 that p only if A at t_2 is psychologically linked, by memory or in some other way, to A at t_1. And as the example is designed to point out, the condition of psychological linking is necessary even if A at t_1 and A at t_2 are the same biological organism.

16. H. Tristram Engelhardt, Jr., "Viability and the Use of the Fetus," in Bondeson, et al., p. 184.

17. Singer, p. 122.

18. Tooley, pp. 411–412.

19. Warren, p. 227.

20. The utilitarian assault of Singer on our intuitions regarding the personhood of all humanity and the nonpersonhood of all other life forms is intense. "To think that the lives of infants are of special value because infants are small and cute is on a par with thinking that a baby seal, with its soft white fur coat and large round eyes deserves greater protection than a whale, which lacks those attributes. Nor can the helplessness or the innocence of the infant *homo sapiens* be a ground for preferring it to the equally helpless and innocent fetal *homo sapiens*, or, for that matter, to laboratory rats who are 'innocent' in exactly the same sense as the human infant, and, in view of the experimenter's power over them, almost as helpless" (pp. 123–124).

   Since newborn human infants are not persons the standard reasons against killing them, in Singer's view, do not apply. Why? Because a policy that permitted infanticide would not threaten anyone capable of understanding it (i.e., since one knows, one would have greater protection than a newborn); a newborn can't conceive of itself as a being with or without a future, and thus can't desire to continue living; a newborn is not autonomous (capable of making decisions) and thus killing it would not violate the principle of respect for persons (pp. 131–138).

21. Singer, pp. 131–138.

22. Tooley, pp. 407–412.

23. Ibid, pp. 411–412.

24. H. Tristram Engelhardt, Jr., "Ethical Issues in Aiding the Death of Young Children," in *Beneficent Euthanasia*, edited by Marvin Kohl, (Buffalo, N.Y.: Prometheus Books, 1975), p. 183.

25. Ibid.

26. Engelhardt, "Viability and the Use of the Fetus," in Bondeson, et al., p. 186.

27. Ibid., p. 190.

28. For a detailed analysis of the concept of persons in the strict sense and the notion of the moral community as it is utilized here, see H. Tristram Engelhardt, Jr., *The Foundations of Bioethics* (New York: Oxford University Press, 1985). According to Engelhardt, the minimum concept of the moral community as a community held together on a basis other than force requires mutual respect by those entities who can conceive of and understand the moral life. Only such entities have moral problems and are objects of unqualified moral respect. The structure of such a broad moral community is found in its procedural agreements, and concrete and relative views of the good life are variously fashioned, discovered, and pursued by particular moral subcommunities and particular moral agents. The life of a particular moral community in a pluralism is justified insofar as it meets the following characteristics: (1) there is mutual respect for the freedom of moral agents; (2) moral controversies are resolved by peaceable means; (3) the free consent of moral agents is the basis of authority; and (4) only persons in a strict sense are unqualified members, persons in a social sense are members because of the roles they have in the community.

29. John Fletcher, "Prenatal Diagnosis, Selective Abortion, and the Ethics of Withholding Treatment From the Defective Newborn," in *Genetic Counseling*, edited by A. M. Capron, et al., (New York: Alan R. Liss, Inc., 1979), p. 248.

30. Angela R. Holder, *Legal Issues in Pediatric and Adolescent Medicine* (New York: John Wiley & Sons, 1977), p. 109.

31. Leonard H. Glantz, "The Role of Personhood in Treatment Decisions Made by Courts," *Milbank Memorial Fund Quarterly/Health and Society* 61 (Winter 1983): 76–100.

32. Cf., H. Tristram Engelhardt, Jr., "Clinical Problems and the Concept of Disease," in *Health, Disease, and Causal Explanations in Medicine*, edited by Lennart Nordenfelt and B. Ingemar B. Lindahl, (Dordrecht, Netherlands: D. Reidel Publishing Co., 1984), pp. 27–41. Rulings in such cases as "Baby Doe" and "Baby Jane Doe," involving the nontreatment of neonates with Down syndrome and spina bifida respectively, to be discussed in greater detail in Chapter 7, have gone against the grain of activist groups who advocate genetic-based views of personhood.

33. Cf., Tom L. Beauchamp and James F. Childress, *Principles of Biomedical Ethics*, 2nd. edition (New York: Oxford University Press, 1983), Chapter 4.

34. Jerome A. Shaffer, "Pain and Suffering: Philosophical Perspectives," *Encyclopedia of Bioethics*, p. 1181. The discussion of pain and suffering relies heavily on this source. See also David E. Boeyink, "Pain and Suffering," *Journal of Religious Ethics* 2 (1974): 85–98.

35. The attitude and response to "pain" can be positive, e.g., masochism. Thus one can rationally say "it hurts so good." Pain is not always disvalued. However, this aspect of pain is not of interest here since this sort of interpretation of experience is beyond the capacities of a neonate.

36. Shaffer, p. 1182.

37. I have applied the principle of beneficence to clinical relationships involving adult patients in another volume, see "To Benefit and Respect Persons: A Challenge for Beneficence in Health Care," in *Beneficence and Health Care*, edited by Earl E. Shelp (Dordrecht, Netherlands: D. Reidel Publishing Co., 1982), pp. 199–222.

38. James Rachels, "The Sanctity of Life," in *Biomedical Ethics Review, 1983*, edited by James A. Humber and Robert F. Almeder, (Clifton, N.J.: Humana Press, 1983), p. 36. See also William K. Frankena, "The Ethics of Respect for Life," in *Respect for Life*, by Owsei Temkin, W. K. Frankena, and Sanford H. Kadish (Baltimore, Md.: Johns Hopkins University Press, 1976), pp. 24–62.

39. John J. Paris, S.J., considers an extreme sanctity-of-life approach "foreign to the traditional Christian understanding of life and the duty one has for its care." The duty to care is limited, not requiring "heroic sacrifice and suffering on the part of the individual or the family, but only the use of ordinary means and resources to preserve it." Thus, Paris favors a contextual approach to decisions, one that takes account of multiple factors beyond the condition of the patient. See John J. Paris, "Right to Life Doesn't Demand Heroic Sacrifice," *Wall Street Journal*, November 28, 1983, p. 30.

40. Gerald Kelly, *Medico-Moral Problems* (St. Louis, Mo.: Catholic Hospital Association, 1958), p. 129.

41. Ibid.

42. Ibid., p. 132.

43. Cf., ibid., p. 134.

44. Cf., John P. Reeder, Jr., "Beneficence, Supererogation, and Role Duty," in Shelp, *Beneficence and Health Care*, pp. 83–108.

45. Pope Pius XII articulated the distinction in an address to an international congress of anesthesiologists as follows: "[N]ormally one is held to use only ordinary means [for the preservation of life and health]—according to circumstances of persons, places, times, and culture—that is to say, means that do not involve any grave burden for oneself and others." See S. Bok, "Death and Dying: Euthanasia: Ethical Views," *Encyclopedia of Bioethics*, p. 270. For a discussion of historical sources, distinctions, and applications of "ordinary" and "extraordinary," see Kelly, pp. 128–141; Beauchamp and Childress, pp. 126–136; President's Commission for the Study of Ethical Prob-

lems in Medicine and Biomedical and Behavorial Research, *Deciding to Forego Life-Sustaining Treatment* (Washington, D.C.: U.S. Government Printing Office, 1983), pp.82–89.

46. Cf., Earl E. Shelp, ed., *Theology and Bioethics* (Dordrecht, Netherlands: D. Reidel Publishing Co., 1985).

Chapter 6. To Kill or Let Die

1. Laila Williamson, "Infanticide: An Anthropological Analysis," in *Infanticide and the Value of Life*, edited by Marvin Kohl (Buffalo, N.Y.: Prometheus Books, 1978), p. 61.

2. Ibid., p. 62.

3. Ibid., p. 61.

4. Ibid., p. 67.

5. Barbara A. Kellum, "Infanticide in England in the Later Middle Ages," *History of Childhood Quarterly* 1, 376f.

6. Maria W. Piers, *Infanticide Past and Present* (New York: W. W. Norton, 1978), p. 56. Langer and Behlmer, in separate studies, noted an increase in rates of infanticide in Europe during the period of 1750–1850, a period in which European population grew by 100 million and placed, no doubt, a great strain on available resources. Economic factors also have been used to explain the prevalence of infanticide (particularly selective female infanticide) at certain periods in the histories of China, Japan, and India. Cf., William L. Langer, "Checks on Population Growth: 1750–1850," *Scientific American* 226, 2:98; and George K. Behlmer, "Deadly Motherhood: Infanticide and Medical Opinion in Mid-Victorian England," *Journal of the History of Medicine and Allied Sciences* 34 (1979): 405. See also Williamson, p. 68; and William L. Langer, "Further Notes on the History of Infanticide," *History of Childhood Quarterly* 2, 1: 131–133.

7. Williamson, pp. 63, 66.

8. Ibid., p. 65.

9. Kellum, p. 378.

10. Williamson, p. 64.

11. Plato wrote: "[O]ffspring of the good should be nurtured, those of inferior men and women, or 'born defective' will be disposed of secretly." Plato, *Republic* 460c, in *Plato, The Collected Dialogues*, edited by Edith Hamilton and Huntington Cairns (Princeton, N.J.: Princeton University Press, 1961).

12. Aristotle wrote in *Politics:* "[A]s to the exposure and rearing of children, let there be a law that no deformed child shall live. . . . ''

Aristotle, *Politics*, translated by Benjamin Jowett, (Oxford: Clarendon Press, 1916), Book 7, Chapter 16.

13. Seneca compared infanticide of a defective infant with putting sickly sheep to the knife "to keep them from infecting the flock." Seneca, *Moral Essays*, translated by John W. Basore, (London: W. Heinemann, Ltd., 1928), p. 145.

14. Plutarch, writing about the practice in Sparta, explained that deformed infants were exposed "in the conviction that the life of that which nature had not well equipped at the very beginning through health and strength was of no advantage either to itself or to the state." Plutarch, *Lives*, 16.2.

15. Owsei Temkin, trans., *Soranus' Gynecology* (Baltimore, Md.: Johns Hopkins University Press, 1956), pp. 79–80.

16. According to Haffter, the advice given to parents included the following: "One must treat their child so badly that they [the demon parents] felt sorry for it and came to fetch it. It must be exposed at a crossroads at midnight or on the beach of the water whence it came. In certain places it must be beaten nine times with birch rods until it bled while the parents called out: 'Take yours and bring me mine!' One should hold it over boiling water and threaten to plunge it in. The oven should be heated with nine different kinds of wood and the child placed on the shovel as if it was intended to thrust it into the fire. The child should be placed on the red-hot shovel, passed into red-hot ashes, laid on a red-head grid, shots should be fired over it, it should be fed on leather and red-hot iron, it should be given poison to drink." Carl Haffter, "The Changeling: History and Psychodynamics of Attitudes to Handicapped Children in European Folklore," *Journal of History of Behavioral Sciences* 4 (1968): 57. See also the relevant sections in Chapter 2 of this volume.

17. For a general discussion of popular causative explanations for the birth of a deformed newborn, see Barbara K. Greenleaf, *Children Through the Ages* (New York: McGraw-Hill, 1978), pp. 48–52; Haffter, "The Changeling"; and Robert Weir, *Selective Nontreatment of Handicapped Newborns* (New York: Oxford University Press, 1984), p.19.

18. deMause, p. 27.

19. Williamson, p. 68.

20. Ibid.; also Greenleaf, p. 19.

21. Williamson, pp. 65f.

22. Ibid., p. 63; also Piers, p. 63.

23. Williamson, p. 64.

24. Greenleaf, p. 19. An example of this claiming of an infant is the

Athenian custom of Amphidromia, a family ceremony somewhat akin to christening. The newborn was placed at the father's feet usually within one week of birth. If he held the child, it was allowed to live, named before the assembled family, and taken into it. If the father refused to pick up the child, turning away from it, "a slave was dispatched to carry the infant from the house and [to] get rid of it. The methods chosen varied from throwing babies into rivers to flinging them into dung heaps and 'potting' them in jars." Prior to the performance of the rite, infants could be exposed with impunity. After the rite and acceptance into the family, if a father killed a child he was subject only to legal charges if brought by a family member. The Greek state could not initiate the charge. Glanville Williams, "The Legal Evaluation of Infanticide," in Kohl, p. 116; and R. H. Feen, "Abortion and Exposure in Ancient Greece: Assessing the Status of the Fetus and 'Newborn' From Classical Sources," in *Abortion and the Status of the Fetus,* edited by W. B. Bondeson, et al., (Dordrecht, Netherlands: D. Reidel Publishing Co., 1983), p. 287.

25. Williamson, p. 64.
26. For example, Augustine, "On the Merits and Remission of Sins and on the Baptism of Infants," Book I, Chapter 28, *Nicene and Post-Nicene Fathers of the Christian Church* V, edited by Philip Schaff (Grand Rapids, Mich.: William B. Eerdmans Publishing Co., 1971), p. 25. Far from entertaining the possibility of reincarnation, medieval Christendom saw the dead infant's soul as, at best, eternally consigned to limbo. Thus, the killing of an infant was officially regarded during the medieval period as much more serious than the killing of older humans. Older humans conceivably would have had an opportunity to be baptized; the dead infant would not.
27. Kellum, p. 369.
28. Williams, p. 118.
29. An English physician, Charles Mercier, expressed this view in 1911 in the following words: "In comparison with other cases of murder, a minimum of harm is done by it. . . . The victim's mind is not sufficiently developed to enable it to suffer from the contemplation of approaching suffering or death. It is incapable of feeling fear or terror. Nor is its consciousness sufficiently developed to enable it to suffer pain in appreciable degree. Its loss leaves no gap in any family circle, deprives no children of their breadwinner or their mother, no human being of a friend, helper or companion. The crime diffuses no sense of insecurity. No one feels a whit less safe because the crime has been committed. It is a racial crime, purely and solely. Its ill effect is not on society as it is, but in striking at the provision of future citizens, to take the place of those who are growing old; and

by whose loss in the course of nature, the community must dwindle and die out, unless it is replenished by the birth and upbringing of children.'' Cited by Glanville Williams in Kohl p. 118.

30. Piers, pp. 48ff.
31. deMause, pp. 26, 28; Feen, pp. 287–288; and Greenleaf, p. 19.
32. William L. Langer, ''Infanticide: A Historical Survey,'' *History of Childhood Quarterly* 1, 3:354.
33. Greenleaf, p. 19. Greenleaf cites a passage from Seneca's ''controversy'' in which the practice is defended: ''Look on the blind wandering about the streets leaning on their sticks, and those with crushed feet, and still again look on those with broken limbs. This one is without arms, that one has had its shoulders pulled down out of shape in order that his grotesqueries may excite laughter. . . . Let us go to the origin of all those ills—a laboratory for the manufacture of human wrecks—a cavern filled with the limbs torn from living children. . . . What wrong has been done to the Republic? On the contrary, have not these children been done a service inasmuch as their parents had cast them out?''
34. Piers, p. 68; also Mary Martin McLaughlin, ''Survivors and Surrogates: Children and Parents From the Ninth to the Thirteenth Centuries,'' in Lloyd deMause, pp. 120–121.
35. Behlmer, p. 410; see also William Blackstone, *Commentaries on the Laws of England*, Vol. 4 (Chicago: University of Chicago Press, 1979), p. 198.
36. Piers, p. 68.
37. Ibid., p. 54.
38. Langer, ''Infanticide: A Historical Survey,'' p. 360.
39. Piers, p. 56.
40. Ibid., pp. 66–67.
41. Langer, ''Checks on Population Growth: 1750–1850,'' p. 98. The institutions of the professional wet nurse and the foundling home grew especially rapidly during the eighteenth and nineteenth centuries in Europe, partly in response to a dramatic rise in the frequency of illegitimate pregnancies. This increase in illegitimacy, in turn, can be explained by a number of powerful social forces. Langer, ''Infanticide: A Historical Survey,'' p. 357.

   Among the most significant social forces that increased illegitimate pregnancies were: (a) large migrations of people, male and female, from rural areas to large cities as a result of economic pressures created by the Industrial Revolution; (b) the upset of traditional marriage patterns by these migrations; (c) the need, on the part of unmarried women, to secure employment—usually either as domestic or as factory workers—in order to survive; (d) the sexual exploitation of such women by their male employers, a practice which became so widespread that, especially in France and England, sexual favors were commonly looked on as practical requirements for continued employment; (e) a reduction in the supply of marriageable men brought about by the maintenance of large, standing armies, and by military incentives for soldiers to remain unmarried; and (f) in response to (e), a great increase in the numbers of unmarried women, particularly rural women, engaged in prostitution in areas adjacent to military encampments. Cf., Williamson, p. 69; Langer, "Infanticide: A Historical Survey," p. 357; and Piers, pp.60–61.

42. Joseph Gallagher, trans., "Fostering the Nobility of Marriage and the Family," *The Documents of Vatican II* (New York: Corpus Books, 1966), p. 256.

43. Cf., Leo Alexander, "Medical Science Under Dictatorship," *New England Journal of Medicine* 241 (July 14, 1949): 39–47.

44. William A. Silverman, "Mismatched Attitudes About Neonatal Death," *Hastings Center Report* 11 (December 1981): 13.

45. See, for example, John A. Robertson, "Involuntary Euthanasia of Defective Newborns: A Legal Analysis," *Stanford Law Review* 27 (January 1975): 213–269, esp. p. 217.

46. See Harold F. Moore, "Acting and Refraining," *Encyclopedia of Bioethics* (New York: Macmillan–Free Press, 1978), pp. 32–38. More precisely, the nonmoral component focuses on human agency and distinguishes between two types of events and/or processes in the world: (a) those that result from the intentional, voluntary movements of a person's body and, in the absence of those movements, would not have occurred, other things being equal; and (b) those that come about independently of the intentional, voluntary movements of a person's body, in some sense independently requiring further articulation. Events of type (a) are the results of human doing (acting, action, etc.), while those of type (b) *may* be the results of human refraining (omitting, letting happen, etc.). The precise requirements for an event of type (b) to count as an instance of human refraining are subject to dispute, but they usually include such factors as: The human properly described as refraining must be aware of the event in question, must be in a position to do something that would alter the event, and, among other things, must have formed an intention *not* so to alter.

47. E.g., Jonathan Glover, *Causing Death and Saving Lives* (New York: Penguin Books, 1977); and Jonathan Bennett, "Whatever the Consequences," *Analysis* 26 (1966): 83–102.

48. E.g., Raziel Abelson, "To Do or Let Happen," *American Philosophical*

Quarterly 19 (July 1982): 219–228; and Daniel Dinello, "On Killing and Letting Die," *Analysis* 31 (1971): 83–86.

49. For while, on the one hand, it is true that the doing/refraining distinction may not yet have been refined to the point that there are *no* cases which it fails to decide, it is also true, on the other hand, that the application of the distinction to a broad range of cases *is* clear. Few concepts, if any, are without their penumbra of vagueness—i.e., cases in which the application of a concept is uncertain. In this respect, then, the doing/refraining distinction is not markedly different from many other concepts that serve well enough, both in everyday life and in science.

50. It might be objected that this statement of the principle is already slanted too much in the direction of utilitarianism by the phrases "bring about evil" and "prevent a like evil", where "evil" is understood to denote evil states of affairs. If so, the principle could be revised: Wrongful action is morally more serious than wrongful omission, given equivalent gravity of resulting consequences. Here "wrongful" is neutral as between deontological wrongs and utilitarian wrongs.

51. Cf., Peter Singer, "Unsanctifying Life," in *Ethical Issues Relating to Life and Death*, edited by John Ladd (New York: Oxford University Press, 1979), pp. 41–61.

52. At least they are *apparent* wrong-making characteristics, in the sense that their presence would serve to elicit a more negative intuitive moral evaluation from most people, other things being equal.

53. Raziel Abelson attempts to defend the doing/refraining distinction by denying that six external features [(1) gravity of foreseeable harm; (2) viciousness of motive; (3) subjective certainty of result; (4) effort, risk, and/or sacrifice required of not acting or not refraining; (5) premeditation; and (6) special responsibility of culprit toward victim] suffice for the moral evaluation of actions. He claims that, in addition to these, there are three other features that are *internal* to actions (i.e., possessed by *all* actions and by *no* omissions) and always bear in a negative way on the moral evaluation of actions. From this it would follow that, whenever an action and an omission are equally seriously wrong on all other scores, the action will be *more* seriously wrong than the omission because of the presence in the action of the three *internal* wrong-making features.

Abelson's arguments, however, constitute no serious challenge to the claims defended in this volume since they either are highly questionable in themselves or simply fail to apply to the types of case with which this volume is concerned. As an example of the former, consider Abelson's claim that susceptibility to precise dating is an internal feature of actions. Presumably, since actions are events, we can tell precisely *when* they have occurred; but since omissions are not events, we are in a greater state of ignorance about when an omission has "occurred." To show the implausibility of this claim in its most general form a single case will suffice. A man walking by a pond notices a child struggling in the water near the shore. The man considers saving the child, but is concerned that he would thereby ruin his new suit of clothes. So the man walks by, leaving the child to drown. Abelson claims that, since the man's omission is not an event, we cannot tell exactly when the omission occurred. But indeed we can define an *interval*, beginning with the moment at which the man first became aware of the child's plight and ending with the moment at which resuscitation became impossible, during which the man's act of saving was morally required. It then follows that the omission in question occurred *during* this interval. Thus it appears that susceptibility to precise dating is not an internal feature of actions as Abelson claims, since it can be possessed by omissions as well.

As examples of Abelson's claims that, even if true in themselves, yet fail to apply to the types of case dealt with in this volume, consider the following. First, Abelson claims that evil actions contain a passive component that is morally equivalent to a fully culpable omission. This is so, he thinks, because once we have initiated a causal chain through our evil action, we must, if the chain is to run to completion, stand back and *let* the evil we have initiated take place. But surely, Abelson argues, if the action itself is evil, then the action *plus* the passive component morally equivalent to a fully culpable omission is morally *worse* than an otherwise comparably evil omission *simpliciter*. That this point, even if true, fails to apply in cases of accelerating the deaths of severely defective newborns becomes obvious when we recall that, in regard to such newborns, the decision has already been made that it *is* morally permissible to allow them to die. Thus the omission involved in such cases is not morally culpable, and therefore the *action* of accelerating death in such cases can contain no passive component morally equivalent to a fully culpable omission.

A second example of the inapplicability of Abelson's arguments to the kinds of case discussed here is his claim that all evil actions involve the violation of a strict moral duty, whereas any evil omission involves merely the violation of a nonstrict moral duty. Together with his claim that violations of strict duties are per se worse than violations of nonstrict duties, it follows that evil actions are per se worse than evil omissions. This point, even if true, cannot bear on cases involving accelerated death of severely defective newborns. For the moral duties about which Abelson speaks must be interpreted as duties owed to *persons*, in the full moral sense of the term. But as I have argued in Chapter 5, it is incorrect to regard a newborn infant as a person in the full moral sense. Thus, Abelson's argument from the relative strictness of duties establishes nothing about the relative seriousness, in the case of a severely defective newborn, of killing versus letting die.

54. Robert Veatch, *Death, Dying, and the Biological Revolution* (New Haven, Conn.: Yale University Press, 1976), p. 90.

55. Glover, pp. 104f. and 111. His criticisms of these arguments, which differ from the ones offered here, are given on pp. 105–107 and 111–112.

56. Cf., Michael Tooley's formulation of the Moral Symmetry Principle, Michael Tooley, *Abortion and Infanticide* (New York: Oxford University Press, 1983), p. 186.

57. Ibid., p. 187.

58. Veatch, p. 90.

59. The act-omission distinction, while analytically unsatisfactory, seems to serve purposes other than conceptual clarity. For example, the President's Commission for the Study of Ethical Problems in Medicine and Biomedical and Behavioral Research endorsed it because: (1) it is "useful in facilitating acceptance of sound decisions that would otherwise meet unwarranted resistance"; (2) it "serves [through law] as a public affirmation of the high value accorded to each human life"; (3) a "prohibition of active killing helps to produce the correct decision in the great majority of cases"; and (4) "weakening the legal prohibition [based on the distinction] to allow a deliberate taking of life in extreme circumstances would risk allowing wholly unjustified taking of life in less extreme circumstances." *Deciding to Forego Life-Sustaining Treatment* (Washington, D.C.: U.S. Government Printing Office, 1983), pp. 71–72.

60. John M. Freeman, "To Treat or Not to Treat," in *Practical Management of Meningomyelocele* (Baltimore, Md.: University Park Press, 1974), p. 14.

61. Ibid., p. 21.

62. John Lorber, "Early Results of Selective Treatment of Spina Bifida Cystica," *British Medical Journal* 4 (1973): 204.

63. Raymond S. Duff and A. G. M. Campbell, "On Deciding the Care of Severely Handicapped or Dying Persons," in *Intervention and Reflection*, edited by R. Munson (Belmont, Calif.: Wadsworth Publishing Co., 1979), p. 120.

64. Ibid., p. 121.

65. The views of John D. Arras are close to those presented here. Cf., "Toward an Ethic of Ambiguity," *Hastings Center Report* 14 (April 1984): 25–33.

66. Since this mother was not legally emancipated, according to state law, the maternal grandparents had legal authority regarding the infant's medical care.

67. Brand Blanshard, "Wisdom," *Encyclopedia of Philosophy,* Vol. 8 (New York: Macmillan, 1967), p. 322.

Chapter 7. Parental Authority and Public Policy

1. John E. Pless, "The Story of Baby Doe," *New England Journal of Medicine* 309 (September 15, 1983): 664; and Pierson, Ball, and Dowd, Attorneys-at-Law, "Legal Update: Recent Governmental Action Regarding the Treatment of Seriously Ill Newborns," unpublished report dated March 16, 1984, from a law firm advising the American Academy of Pediatrics.

2. Section 504 states, "no otherwise qualified handicapped individual . . . shall, solely by reason of his handicap, be excluded from participation in, be denied the benefits of, or be subjected to discrimination under any program or activity receiving Federal financial assistance. . . ."

3. The full text of the Notice is reproduced in *Hastings Center Report* 12 (August 1982): 6. All subsequent quotes from the Notice are from this source.

4. Norman Fost, "Putting Hospitals on Notice," *Hastings Center Report* 12 (August 1982): 5.

5. Ibid., p. 5.

6. Ibid., pp. 6–7.

7. Ibid., p. 7.

8. Ibid.

9. 48 Fed. Reg. 9630–32 (March 7, 1983).

10. Ibid., 9630.

11. Ibid., 9631.

12. Ibid., 9632.

13. Ibid., 9630.

14. Ibid.

15. Ibid., 9631.

16. *American Academy of Pediatrics* v. *Heckler,* 561 F. Supp. 395 (1983), 398–399. Cf., George J. Annas, "Disconnecting the Baby Doe Hotline," *Hastings Center Report* 13 (June 1983): 14–16.

17. *American Academy of Pediatrics* v. *Heckler*, p. 399.

18. Ibid., p. 395.

19. Ibid., p. 399.

20. Ibid., p. 400.

21. Ibid., p. 401.

22. Ibid., p. 400.

23. 48 Fed. Reg. 30846–52 (July 5, 1983).

24. Ibid., 30851.

25. George J. Annas, "Baby Doe Redux: Doctors as Child Abusers," *Hastings Center Report* 13 (October 1983): 27.

26. 48 Fed. Reg. 30851.

27. Ibid., 30852.

28. Ibid.

29. Ibid.

30. Ibid.

31. Angela R. Holder, "Parents, Courts, and Refusal of Treatment," *Journal of Pediatrics* 103 (October 1983): 519.

32. Annas, "Baby Doe Redux," p. 27.

33. Cf., 49 Fed. Reg. 1623–50 (January 12, 1984).

34. "Comments of the American Academy of Pediatrics on Proposed Rule Regarding Nondiscrimination on the Basis of Handicap Relating to Health Care for Handicapped Infants," reprinted in *Bioethics Reporter* 3 (February 1984), Literature 31–90.

35. Cf., James E. Strain, "The American Academy of Pediatrics Comments on the 'Baby Doe II' Regulations," *New England Journal of Medicine* 309 (August 18, 1983): 444. The government's versions of these investigations are contained in its response to comments published with the final rules in the Federal Register, January 12, 1984, p. 1647. In all, forty-nine investigations are summarized.

36. American Academy of Pediatrics, Committee on Bioethics, "Treatment of Critically Ill Newborns," *Pediatrics* 72 (October 1983): 565–566.

37. Ibid., p. 565.

38. President's Commission for the Study of Ethical Problems in Medicine and Biomedical and Behavioral Research, *Deciding to Forego Life-Sustaining Treatment* (Washington, D.C.: U.S. Government Printing Office, 1983). Chapter 6 is devoted to "Seriously Ill Newborns." Within a review of current decision-making practices, the Commission identified three types of shortcomings: "[1] appropriate information may not be communicated to all those involved in the decision; [2] professionals as well as parents do not at times un-

derstand the bases of a decision to treat or not to treat; and [3] actions can be taken without the informed approval of parents or other surrogates" (p. 209). The tone of the report suggests that these are innocent failings, partially attributable to the circumstances, partially attributable to a failure to identify and evaluate reasons for decisions, and partially attributable to psychological factors related to the assumption of responsibility.

The Commission proposed a "net benefit" standard for treatment decisions. Net benefit was recognized as a "somewhat subjective and imprecise" standard, but considered a "very strict standard." The Commission explains that (1) "net benefit is absent only if the burdens imposed on the patient by the disability or its treatment would lead a competent decision-maker to choose to forego the treatment"; (2) the standard "excludes honoring idiosyncratic views that might be allowed if a person were deciding about his or her own treatment"; (3) the estimate of net benefit, to the extent possible, should be from the infant's own perspective; and (4) the standard "excludes consideration of the negative effects of an impaired child's life on other persons, including parents, siblings, and society" (pp. 218–219).

Infants for whom the net benefit of treatment is unclear or ambiguous pose the greatest difficulty in decision making. Proposals to achieve some consistency in these cases by adopting certain "objective" criteria that separate treatable infants from nontreatable infants are rejected as being shown not to improve the quality of decision making in this category of infants. As noted in the text of this chapter, the Commission endorsed a review procedure utilizing ethics committees as a means to enhance the quality of decisions in these ambiguous cases.

The Commission saw a moral link between decisions to sustain the life of a seriously ill neonate and the duty to "provide the continuing care that makes a reasonable range of life choices possible" (p. 228). This may mean increased funding for support programs that supplement the limited resources of individual families to provide "humane continuing care," provisions for adoption and foster care of these children, and emotional and other support for parents who bear the burden of care. The Commission realized that these services and the assurance of adequate care for the rescued infant may require public funding, without which society's "moral authority to intervene on behalf of a newborn whose life is in jeopardy is compromised" (p. 229).

39. American Academy of Pediatrics, "Treatment of Critically Ill Newborns," p. 566. Cf., American Academy of Pediatrics, Infant Bioeth-

ics Task Force and Consultants, "Guidelines for Infant Bioethics Committees," *Pediatrics* 74 (August 1984): 306–310.

40. 49 Fed. Reg. 1623.

41. 49 Fed Reg. 1622–1654, esp. pp. 1650–1654.

42. Ibid., 1651.

43. Ibid.

44. Ibid., 1652.

45. *United States of America* v. *University Hospital, State U. of New York at Stony Brook,* CA. No. 83–6343 (2d Cir. Feb. 23, 1984), 1905.

46. George J. Annas, "The Case of Baby Jane Doe: Child Abuse or Unlawful Federal Intervention?" *American Journal of Public Health* 74 (July 1984): 727.

47. *In the Matter of William E. Weber, Guardian Ad Litem for Baby Jane Doe* v. *Stony Brook Hospital, et al.,* CA. No. 672 (Court of Appeals, N.Y., October 28, 1983).

48. *United States of America* v. *University Hospital, State U. of New York at Stony Brook,* CV. 83–4818 (U.S. Dist Ct., Eastern District of New York, November 17, 1983).

49. *United States of America* v. *University Hospital, State U. of New York at Stony Brook,* CA. No. 83–6343 (2d Cir. February 23, 1984).

50. Ibid., pp. 1923–1924.

51. Ibid., p. 1929.

52. *American Hospital Assn., etc.* v. *Margaret M. Heckler,* and *American Medical Assn., et al.* v. *Margaret M. Heckler,* 585 F. Supp. 541 (1984).

53. Congressional Record, September 19, 1984, H 9806.

54. 49 Fed. Reg. 48160–73 (December 10, 1984).

55. Infant is a baby less than one year of age unless born extremely premature, or hospitalized since birth, or with long-term disabilities. Ibid., 48166.

56. Ibid., 48162.

57. Reasonable medical judgment is that which is medically indicated according to "a reasonably prudent physician, knowledgeable about the case and the treatment possibilities with respect to the medical conditions involved. It is not to be based on subjective 'quality of life' or other abstract concepts." Ibid., 48163.

58. Ibid., 48164.

59. Ibid.

60. Ibid., 49162.

61. Ibid., 48172.

62. Ibid., 48171.

63. 50 Fed. Reg. 14878-14901 (April 15, 1985).

64. Ibid., 14880.

65. Editorial, "'Baby Doe' Legislation Creates More Problems," *American Medical News* 27 (August 10, 1984): 4.

66. Michael Wald, "State Intervention on Behalf of 'Neglected' Children: A Search for Realistic Standards," *Stanford Law Review* 27 (April 1975): 993.

67. Phyllis S. Glick, et al., "Pediatric Nursing Homes," *New England Journal of Medicine* 309 (September 15, 1983): 640–646.

68. 59 Am Jur 2d, Parent and Child, p. 98.

69. John A. Robertson, "Discretionary Non-Treatment of Defective Newborns," in *Genetics and the Law,* edited by Aubrey Milunsky and George J. Annas (New York: Plenum Press, 1976), p. 458.

70. *In Re Hofbauer,* 419 N.Y. 2d 940–941. The opinion states:

> What constitutes adequate medical care . . . cannot be judged in a vacuum free from external influences, but rather each case must be decided on its own particular facts. . . . This inquiry [regarding an eight-year-old with Hodgkin's disease] cannot be posed in terms of whether the parent has made a "right" or a "wrong" decision, for the present state of the practice of medicine despite its vast advances, very seldom permits such definitive conclusions. Nor can a court assume the role of a surrogate parent and establish as the objective criteria with which to evaluate a parent's decision its own judgment as to the exact method or degree of medical treatment which should be provided, for such standard is fraught with subjectivity. Rather, in our view, the court's inquiry should be whether the parents, once having sought accredited medical assistance and having been made aware of the seriousness of their child's affliction and the possibility of a cure if a certain mode of treatment is undertaken, have provided for their child a treatment which is recommended by their physician and which has not been totally rejected by all responsible medical authority.

71. Angela R. Holder, *Legal Issues in Pediatrics and Adolescent Medicine* (New York: John Wiley & Sons, 1977), pp. 114–115; and John A. Robertson, "Involuntary Euthanasia of Defective Newborns: A Legal Analysis," *Stanford Law Review* 27 (January 1975): 213–269.

72. I am indebted to Raymond Duff for helping me to understand this more clearly.

Index